Dr Álvaro Campi

The Truth About
The Dukan Diet

Discover why Dukan is the
healthy way to lose weight

**HODDER &
STOUGHTON**

First published in Great Britain in 2013 by Hodder & Stoughton
An Hachette UK company

1

Copyright © Dr Álvaro Campillo Soto 2013

The right of Dr Álvaro Campillo Soto to be identified as the
Author of the Work has been asserted by him in accordance
with the Copyright, Designs and Patents Act 1988.

A CIP catalogue record for this title is available from the British Library

Trade Paperback ISBN 978 1 444 77685 0
Ebook ISBN 978 1 444 77686 7

Translated by Morag Jordan

Typeset in Celeste by Hewer Text UK Ltd, Edinburgh

Printed and bound by Clays Ltd, St Ives plc

Hodder & Stoughton policy is to use papers that are natural, renewable
and recyclable products and made from wood grown in sustainable
forests. The logging and manufacturing processes are expected to
conform to the environmental regulations of the country of origin.

Hodder & Stoughton Ltd
338 Euston Road
London NW1 3BH
www.hodder.co.uk

To Leticia, who is my whole life
To my parents, for everything

Contents

Contents

Contents

Contents

Contents

1.

Why I wrote this book

First of all, I would like start off by introducing myself: my name is Álvaro Campillo Soto. I hold a European Doctorate in medicine and surgery and I work as a consultant in general and digestive surgery at the Morales Meseguer Hospital in Murcia, Spain. I am qualified in applied research methodology for obesity. For two years (2008–2010), I was one of three Spanish doctors who took part in the 'European Obesity Academy' project run by the Karolinska Institute in Stockholm, which awards the Nobel prizes. Working on this project, we helped to greatly develop scientific methodology relating to obesity, as well as designing and carrying out studies on obese patients. It is because of this commitment and this extremely specific experience that I set about writing this book. Furthermore, I received an honourable mention in the Barea awards (the Signo Foundation in Madrid gives these to medical projects) and the Pfizer prize for clinical excellence for my work in the bariatric unit at the hospital where I practise. Also, although I am not overweight or obese at the moment, this has not always been the case; for me, maintaining a healthy weight requires a lot of effort and daily exercise, and I have to give up certain little pleasures too as far as I can. For all these reasons, I like to keep abreast of everything to do with diets and nutrition in general, if only to improve as much as I can the lives of my patients, and of my family and friends who are happy to heed my advice.

Over the past years, the Dukan Diet has been amazingly successful. Lots of people have tried it, everyone from celebrities to the local shopkeeper. It has garnered much criticism as well as praise. I have tested it myself (I like trying things out to see the effects and the drawbacks, to know whether or not I can recommend them). I had stayed on the sidelines of the debate about whether the diet is good or bad for your health, and everything that follows on from this, until recently when I came across the weekly programme *Taller de Salud* (*Health Workshop*), on a local TV channel. That day the episode was devoted to 'The Dukan Diet – lies and truths' and I was horrified by the number of untruths, the absurdity of the ridiculous arguments and the lack of scientific rigour. Taking part were an endocrinologist and a GP, regular contributors to the programme, and on this occasion they were joined by a dietitian and the chairman of the Order of Dietitians and Nutritionists for the region of Murcia. All these experts seemed to know nothing (or pretended to know nothing) about the many studies that have been published which confirm the Dukan Diet's positive effects on health. Very quickly, given all the nonsense being voiced, lots of people who had followed the diet rang into the TV station. Some were worried about what might happen to them, others were frightened out of their wits. Because there wasn't the slightest mention of anything positive about the diet, absolutely nothing at all.

My indignation stayed with me throughout the night; I hardly slept a wink and got up several times. The following morning I felt just as indignant, and outraged by the bias and lack of ethics with which health topics are sometimes tackled. So I read up about the subject again before sending the email below to the head of VerdadTV, to the director of programming as well as to the programme's director and presenter:

> I am writing to you to express my indignation concerning what was said about the Dukan Diet on the *Taller de Salud* programme yesterday. Whether I am for or against this sort of diet is immaterial ; what is intolerable is to go around proclaiming alleged truths simply 'because it's me who says so!', which is what happened on yesterday's programme.
>
> Based on what scientists currently know, not only has it been proved that ketogenic [very low-carbohydrate] and low-carbohydrate diets ARE NOT bad for our health but, as many studies on the subject published in recent years have confirmed (I'll provide you with some references at the end of this message), it has been proved that they have potentially beneficial effects on fat and cardiovascular status: they lower blood pressure, they lower bad cholesterol (LDL [low density lipoprotein]) by increasing good cholesterol (HDL [high

density lipoprotein]) without causing osteoporosis, etc. Yet despite this, on yesterday's programme, Dr Madrid [an endocrinologist and consultant in nutrition at the university hospital of Murcia], set about discrediting these diets, without any scientific arguments or reasoning based on recent scientific publications. In fact, even the diagrams he used to explain how ketogenesis works were inaccurate (you can check this by looking at basic biochemistry texts such as Keith Fryan's work on controlling metabolism).

Some of the arguments that Dr Madrid used were particularly rich, especially these ones: *'In France, 80 per cent of people who have done the Dukan Diet have regained their initial weight after five years'* and *'A friend asked me if he should do the diet and my answer to him was: Would you recommend it to your children? . . . That says it all!'* I am not disputing that if you fail to follow the stabilization advice that you have to apply every week, then you will put weight back on with this diet. But the fact of the matter is, as Dr Madrid must be well aware, that with the other diets (those he describes as healthy) this weight goes back on in just under two years and for 95 per cent of people! Ketogenic diets may not be a cure-all (although based on the figure of 80 per cent that Dr Madrid cites they have a 15 per cent higher success rate) but, at any rate, they are no worse than so-called 'healthy' diets. Not to mention that almost 50 per cent of the people living in the Murcia region are either overweight or obese – which would lead one to believe that the lifestyle advocated by Dr Madrid and his colleagues is not altogether persuasive.

A study published in 2010 compared the Mediterranean diet, a low-carb diet and the diet recommended by the American Association of Diabetes. It established that only the low-carb diet would improve lipid profile (fat levels in the blood) and control glycaemia. This only goes to show that whatever you say should be backed up by proof and that proclaiming yourself to be an expert does not make you right (I thought that this principle of authority had disappeared along with the Middle Ages). Not a word about this in yesterday's programme!

To my great regret, and unfortunately for all the people suffering from cancer, nothing was said either about the potential beneficial effects of ketogenic diets, like the Dukan Diet, in improving quality of life and blood test results for terminal phase cancer patients, as has been shown in several pilot studies.

As for this 'would you recommend it to your children?', we all know that a glass of wine a day is good for our health. So, Dr Madrid, would you recommend this to your children or to the children who come to see you because they are overweight and have cardiovascular problems? Come on, as the scientists we are (or at least are supposed to be), we have no right to use such simplistic and fallacious arguments to sow confusion in the minds of lay people. However, the best in all of this (which ironically highlights the absurdity of the question '*would you recommend it to your children?*') is that ketogenic diets such as the Dukan Diet are successfully prescribed to epileptic children who show resistance to medication. The parents of these children are only too happy to recommend ketogenic diets to their offspring!

We doctors often make the mistake of believing ourselves to be very learned. Without consulting current scientific sources, we base our ideas on acquired knowledge that has been superseded many times. We rely upon a certain magical idea or on arguments drawn from what we thought we had learnt about physiology at medical school. It is not me who says this; time and again this has all been suggested by prestigious researchers, such as Daniel Kahneman, the Nobel Prize winner, Gerd Gigerenzer, the German researcher, Amós Tversky and the whole heuristics and biases school. This sort of attitude leads to confusion among patients and the general public, and even among other doctors who are not specialists in the discipline concerned. Anxiety and fear are spread quite unjustifiably.

Given such systematic denigration, one may well wonder whether it was in the interests of these guest 'experts' – except for Dr Molina Boix [consultant in internal medicine at the university hospital of Murcia] – to limit this type of diet from spreading as it is likely to deter some patients from coming for consultations, reduce their income and run counter to established health policies (which are very often outmoded or modelled on other countries). In this case, as well as needlessly alarming the general public, as far as scientific content goes yesterday's programme is a matter for shame.

It seems to me that you ought to handle this type of matter more seriously if you wish to continue being a source of information, and not of disinformation and scaremongering for the general public. As Richard Feynman, the physics Nobel Prize winner, humanist, free thinker and brilliant professor, used to say: *'It's all about forcing yourself to be rigorous and provide all the information, whether it be positive or negative, so that each person can judge the value of what they are being offered with complete impartiality instead of giving only impartial information that could influence judgement in one direction or another.'*

What happened after I sent this email? Absolutely nothing! As I received no response and no corrections of any sort were made during the following week's programme, I wrote a letter to the editor of the *La Verdad* newspaper, the parent company of the TV channel, and this was not published either. Given the lack of interest in people's health and the refusal to present anything positive about the Dukan Diet, in particular to avoid the many vested interests of various individuals, I decided to expand the work I had done on bibliographical revision on this topic. I wanted to put forward a truthful, honest and scientific point of view about the current state of scientific knowledge and deal with the following topic: *ketogenic diets and the Dukan Diet, the paradigm and popularity of this type of diet.* I wanted this book to be easy to read and to make sense to everyone, whatever their degree of culture and education. This is why I have structured the book around a series of 50 questions with explanatory answers. To round off, I have written chapters dealing specifically with what science knows today about ketogenesis – the effects of low-carbohydrate, ketogenic diets: since the body cannot directly use ingested sugar to produce energy, it draws upon its fat reserves instead – in diseases such as Alzheimer's, cancer and epilepsy. I have also added a brief explanation about neuropharmacology for this type of diet and I conclude with a list of the published works on this topic that I consulted.

I hope that you get as much enjoyment from reading the book as I did from writing it!

Murcia, 11 November 2011

2.

My own experience of the Dukan Diet

I can remember my parents telling me when I was young that the Atkins type of food combining diet was very bad for your health, that such diets helped you lose weight quickly but that you would put it back on again even more quickly. I grew up with this idea imprinted on my brain. As the years went by and I started to study medicine, I took an interest in everything to do with nutrition whenever I had time to spare.

At the same time as this, my father started to suffer with heart problems. He was given various types of treatment. One day, I was extremely surprised to see him come back full of beans after seeing his cardiologist, a professor at the University of Murcia. He had instructed my father to follow the Atkins diet, which was meant to make him lose weight rapidly so that his weight would not have any negative impact on his health. I didn't understand: how could an eminent cardiologist prescribe such a harmful diet?

Instead of hanging on to ideas that had been drummed into me as a child, without any scientific proof other than my parents' principle of authority, I immersed myself in the available scientific literature and searched for any possible benefits this type of diet might have. My first discovery was a report in the science supplement of the *La Verdad* daily newspaper, written by José Antonio Lozano Teruel, a professor of biochemistry at the University of Murcia. It looked at the Atkins diet, and included the following statement: *'A clinical study, presented at a recent American Association of Cardiology annual conference, shows that this type of diet encourages fat loss and weight loss by increasing instead the proportion of high density lipoproteins, commonly known as "good cholesterol".'*

Afterwards, through using the United States National Health Library, I was able to access many other studies which proved that, far from being dangerous for health, these diets achieved comparatively better results, as it were, than any other type of diet. In fact, they had very positive effects on blood fats as well as on diabetes and controlling glucose levels, but without causing the side effects that hearsay attributed to them.

My dealings with this type of diet reached another level two years ago when I was asked by a retirement home in Cartagena, in the region of Murcia, to organize a weight-loss workshop. When I arrived, I explained how these diets worked to those taking part, giving them both the pros and the cons. I warned them that these diets were much criticized, most of the time by people whose own medical practices would be in danger of suffering a decline in clientele or whose so-called 'miracle slimming products and recipes' would be likely to see a drop in sales. I told them that these smears were not substantiated by any scientific evidence and were based on partisan money issues and economic self-interest. The 20 people who took part in the workshop all lost weight. They learnt how to put right any temporary excesses due to family gatherings, meetings or meals out with fellow retired people. Their spirits were much improved and it was striking how their blood tests stabilized. Some of them were even able to dig out clothes from their wardrobes that had been stored away for many years, barely worn because they had become too small almost the moment they'd been bought. So with minimal expenditure these retired people were able to get dressed up to the nines for their grandchildren's first holy communion, which in a period of austerity is surely much appreciated.

Now I often talk to my patients about Dr Dukan's diet; I tell them about the benefits for losing weight as well as for general health. Many of my patients try the Dukan Diet and come back to let me know that they feel better and are in better shape. What is more, their blood tests prove it. As we'll see throughout this book, and as many of my medical colleagues have also confirmed from observing their own patients, the Dukan type of ketogenic diet really is able to improve health outcomes for people who, for example, suffer from high blood pressure or diabetes (but also from other illnesses such as cancer, rheumatism, and so on.)

Lastly, my recent experience with the Dukan Diet has been quite personal. Although I am not fat, I do like to enjoy myself when I'm with friends; at the weekend I like to go and eat some nice tapas or a paëlla and then drink some cocktails with my wife, my brother and friends. I love travelling and tasting gastronomic delights from around Spain or other countries. However, I also know that to be healthy, having a healthy weight is essential, which is why I take exercise every day. Moreover, once a week, I have a protein-only day, as recommended by Dr Dukan. After Christmas and Easter, in the summer or after a run of sumptuous meals, I do 2–3 consecutive days of proteins over a fortnight. The results are spectacular as I manage to lose the extra half stone or so gained during the holidays in under three weeks by getting rid of fat but not muscle. I know this because I always weigh myself at the chemist using the diagnostic scales that analyse body composition. At the end of last summer, thanks to the pure protein days, I had dropped from 13st 2lb (with 19.9 per cent fat) back down to my normal 12st 8lb (and with just 14.8 per cent fat).

I would like to invite critics of the Dukan Diet, as well as all those experts who are sceptical that a diet like this works, to immerse themselves once again in their medical faculty studies (and even add to them through some ad hoc research of their own). I would ask them to read this book, as they will certainly find it most instructive.

3.

Is the Dukan method a good or a bad diet?

Or how to settle a question and resolve a medical uncertainty

By definition, medicine and health are subject to a certain degree of uncertainty. This uncertainty can be divided into three types:

1. *Our individual medical knowledge (that of each doctor) is limited.* However thorough and in-depth our knowledge, we can never know everything about medicine. We do not have all the answers to the questions and doubts that our patients bring to us. This type of uncertainty can be dealt with through study and continuous professional development.
2. *Overall medical knowledge (of medicine) is limited.* Less than 10 years ago, we still believed that the human genome was made up of over 100,000 genes. We now know that there are in fact only about 30,000. What I want to point out here is that medicine does not have all the answers to the questions

it gets asked. This is partly because it is a very complex, imperfect science which is continually developing. It is also due to the limitations bound up with scientific instrumentation and experimentation. However, although we cannot have an answer for everything, we are able to answer more and more questions. To lessen this uncertainty, we have to keep on making scientific progress, day after day, through talking to patients, experimentation and study.

3. *We have to be able to distinguish between these two types of uncertainty.* If we fail to take into account our own ignorance (first uncertainty) and the limitations of medical knowledge as a whole (second uncertainty), we run the risk of making serious mistakes. Our patients will be badly treated and we will bring about dire adverse effects. These can be avoided if, for example, we are able to admit to ourselves that there is a better treatment that we don't know enough about or that this invasive diagnostic test is not as suitable as we'd thought.

Unfortunately, uncertainty is not discussed with students at medical school. Quite the opposite, as what is cultivated there is what we call 'dogmatic certainty': what we are taught in class is to be used in exams and is deemed to be the absolute truth. As a result, most doctors suffer atrophy of their critical faculties (besides sometimes considering themselves to be geniuses!).You may think that I am going a bit far, but there is no doubt that in the history of medicine this attitude has resulted in some significant errors and catastrophes. So it was that Michel Servetus was burnt at the stake for defending the existence of pulmonary circulation, which was not supposed to exist because Dr Galen had made no mention of it centuries earlier. The only conclusion was that poor old Michel must have been sent by Satan; rather than checking to see if what he said was true, it was much simpler to burn him alive. Good riddance! People could carry on sleeping safely in their beds. Three cheers for dogma, and down with critical judgement! Because of this particular mindset, which remains firmly embedded today, my email to VerdadTV went unanswered. Instead of trying to find out about ketogenic diets, the medical 'experts' preferred to believe that they possessed absolute knowledge, whereas in fact they hadn't the slightest idea about what these diets can do. I imagine they must have said to the presenter, who is not a doctor, to the head of the channel, who is not a doctor, and to the head of programming, who is also not a doctor, that this email was a tissue of lies. They must have cloaked themselves in their status of experts who are supposed to be completely on top of their subject. I recommend you never place your trust in a health professional whose only argument is to tell you that *he is the one who knows the matter*, without any other form of procedure or explanation.

Working as a doctor, my patients share with me, on an almost daily basis, doubts and questions for which I have no immediate answer. As far as doubts are concerned, I have some experience that I will try and share with you so that you can either look for the answers yourselves, or insist that your doctor, nutritionist, dietitian or any other health professional does the same. Since, in reality, when confronted with a question that has no immediate answer three stances are possible:

1. *The easiest stance*, based on what you think you know, involves inventing a theory about the problem under discussion and trying to make it sound as credible as possible. Although very common, this is the most dishonest stance possible and should be banned forever. It is rooted in what is called the 'principle of authority', according to which any words uttered by a person qualified in their field are as such deemed to be the truth. It is this attitude that holds sway among all those people who criticize the Dukan Diet and ketogenic diets in general.

2. *The noblest stance* involves acknowledging our uncertainty and that we do not have any accurate knowledge of the matter (and possibly referring the patient to a colleague who is more qualified in this field).

3. *The most difficult stance* involves searching for the answer by using all available sources of information and cross-referencing the various existing positions so as to arrive at a logical conclusion. Of all of them, this stance is the least commonly adopted as it requires us firstly to recognize that we do not know

(as with the previous stance) and then to devote time and effort to hunting down information that will throw light on the matter for us.

When you have made up your mind to search for the answer yourself, what do you do? If you were approaching this seriously and scrupulously, you would consult the current list of published research on the subject. Nowadays, this is dead easy: all you have to do is go to the Pubmed® website (www.pubmed.com), the freely accessible search engine for the MEDLINE database which contains extracts and article abstracts for biomedical research made available to everyone by the United States National Health Library. This library holds almost 5,000 medical journals and over 20 million listed articles. Whenever you are looking for an answer to a medical query, logic would dictate that you seek it in this library, which offers access to the world's best and most prestigious journals. This is where I go and this is where I searched when examining ketogenic diets and the Dukan Diet, which is where our interest lies.

Clearly, if you type 'Dukan' into the search engine no results will come up, probably because this diet is still too new to have had any studies published about it. However, as the Dukan Diet is one example of ketogenic, high-protein and low-fat, diets we can always search for articles about these diets in general. So I started my research by typing in 'ketogenic diet', which brought up 1,082 articles. Next I typed 'ketogenic diet cancer' (52 articles), 'ketogenic diet epilepsy' (695 articles), 'ketogenic diet weight loss' (88 articles), 'ketogenic diet diabetes' (51 articles), 'ketogenic diet brain' (301 articles) and, lastly, 'ketogenic diet review' (282 articles). I completed my research with the following terms: 'Atkins diet cardiovascular' (147 articles) and 'Atkins diet effects' (394 articles), the Atkins being the best-known ketogenic diet (but with no restriction on fats), the likelihood being that the search engine, based on key words, would list all the articles about ketogenesis under the heading Atkins.

After sifting through these results, I ended up with 244 published studies and articles about the subject which I was then able to review and analyse. This research means that I am able to explain to you here, in simple terms but without lacking any scientific rigour, the truth about this type of diet with the generic name 'ketogenic diets'. As far as I am aware, this book is the most comprehensive scientific work ever undertaken to collate, review, analyse and summarize what is known about this type of diet.

As you will see from the appendix, 'A few letters in reply to "my dear expert" nutritionists, fierce critics of the Dukan Diet', I enjoy writing letters, like Cyrano de Bergerac. So I have answered all the unfounded criticism that I've found in the press by writing letters. If these 'experts' had done their work, they would not have terrified the general public and I would not have felt compelled to write this book – although I have to admit that it has been a pleasure!

In order to make the book easy to follow, I have written the main chapter as a series of 50 very specific questions about the diet and how it can be used in different circumstances and with various illnesses, so that anyone reading it can form a quick but comprehensive idea of what they can expect from the diet in each concrete situation. Furthermore, you will find a very instructive section on neuropharmacology for ketogenic diets, as well as chapters devoted to some of the currently most common pathologies – cancer, Alzheimer's disease, metabolic syndrome (when the metabolism is generally not working properly; it can foreshadow several serious illnesses, such as diabetes or cardiovascular problems), high blood pressure, hypercholesterolaemia, diabetes and heart disease.

To make things easier and more pleasant for you, in addition to an informal style (but nonetheless scientifically rigorous) style I have included a large number of tables, drawings and diagrams throughout the book to help clarify and summarize the questions being dealt with.

4.

50 questions

Or unravelling the truths and lies about the Dukan Diet

1. What is the Dukan Diet? [1-4]

The Dukan Diet is not simply a diet. It is a method that has elements dealing with a) behaviour and society, and b) nutrition and metabolism.

Both these dimensions go hand in hand. However, here we will be looking only at the section on nutrition and metabolism as it is the area that has come under fire and therefore merits scientific light being shed on it.

As far as nutrition is concerned, the Dukan Diet aims to reduce carbohydrate intake and limit fat intake. It allows you to eat 100 foods: 72 foods rich in animal or vegetable proteins, without any particular restriction on quantity, and 28 vegetables that you can eat as much of as you want.

In effect, the Dukan Diet is a high-protein diet that can be related to the ketogenic diet model, about which there is a great deal of scientific literature.

One of the main features of this diet is that it is structured *in four phases* which make it easier to follow the method and get results:

Phase 1 (or the Attack phase): lasts for an average of 4–5 days; you are allowed only the 72 high-protein foods. Weight loss as fat gets burnt up is easy, extremely fast and motivating.

Phase 2 (or the Cruise phase): the pure protein days alternate with days of proteins and vegetables. Weight loss occurs more gradually, making it possible to avoid vitamin and mineral deficiencies, constipation and any monotony from eating only a protein-based diet. In theory, this phase progresses with 2lb (1kg) being lost per week, until you reach your True Weight.

Phase 3 (or the Consolidation phase): this is one of the most important phases in the method; now the diet opens up to include five other food groups, thereby providing a basic eating model that is easy to visualize. It forms a safety platform and barrier to prevent you from falling back into your bad old ways, while you continue to eat as much as before. This is a transitional phase that lasts five days for each pound shed. What is good about it is that it steers you clear of the rebound effect that you get with any type of standard weight-loss diet (the weight that is lost gets put back on again).

Phase 4 (or the Permanent Stabilization phase): after a certain period, the eating model learnt during the Consolidation phase has become well enough embedded; new habits have been adopted and you no longer require supervision about what to eat. Nevertheless, in order to avoid the very many temptations of daily life and address your vulnerability to putting on weight (your initial weight gain was proof of this), the Dukan Diet gets you to stick to three rules that are simple, effective and hardly frustrating, but *non-negotiable* – and which you must follow for the rest of your life!

- A day of proteins every week (on a set day, for example, on Thursdays)
- A daily 20-minute walk, and you never take any lifts or escalators
- Three tablespoons of oat bran every day

Unlike the Atkins diet, where fat intake is unrestricted, the Dukan Diet has a list of no-fat or low-fat foods that you can eat. So with Dukan, weight loss is faster than it is with Atkins. What is more, with Dukan, you are allowed foods such as skimmed milk or 0% fat yoghurt, which makes the diet easier and more agreeable than the Atkins diet (which bans yoghurt and fromage frais).

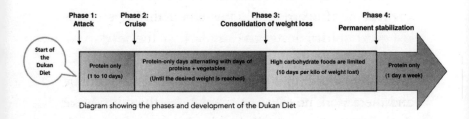

Diagram showing the phases and development of the Dukan Diet

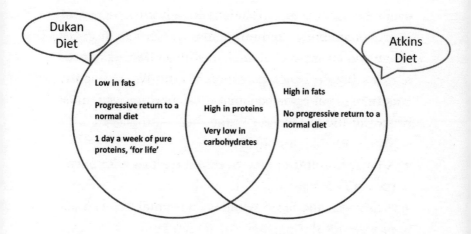

2. How did the ketogenic diet come about? [5–16]

The ketogenic diet was rediscovered by Dr Robert Atkins, who popularized it in the 1970s with his book *Dr Atkins' Diet Revolution*. However, in actual fact the person who officially founded these diets was an obese Englishman called William Banting, who lived in the nineteenth century. In 1863, he published a text about his experience of losing weight using a diet based on lots of meat and fish, but very little bread, fruit and vegetables.

However, if we want to know where this type of diet really comes from we need to look at the lifestyle of prehistoric man: for primitive man, food was scarce, and especially carbohydrates (fruit was not easy to come by, and there were no cakes or sweets). On the other hand, there were molluscs, shellfish, fish, coconuts, earth worms, plant roots (the equivalent of today's vegetables) and a few small animals or carrion. This is how primitive people, who developed what is called a 'thrifty genotype', managed to survive and reproduce, and how their genes got passed down to us. We are the direct descendants of humans whose genotype enabled them to store great quantities of energy, which makes us put on weight easily if we eat a lot, especially if the meals are packed with easily absorbable carbohydrates.

What is this 'thrifty genotype'? Individuals with physiological insulin resistance have this genotype; surplus glucose feeds the brain while at the same time rapidly producing fat during times of food abundance, so that energy reserves are available during periods of food shortage. Insulin is a hormone produced by the pancreas: it controls our blood sugar level (glycaemia) and in particular it turns sugar into energy and fat (energy 'reserves' for later use). With insulin resistance, the insulin has less effect on the sugar which means the sugar continues circulating in the blood without being properly metabolized into energy, which increases glycaemia and the risk of diabetes and leads to a tendency to produce fat.

In prehistoric times, individuals who were able to store energy from sugar (in particular as fat) were at an advantage with regard to survival and reproduction compared to those who could not store this energy. These fat stores were then depleted through the muscles' daily work (walking for long periods, fleeing from danger over several hours, transporting materials, food, etc.). By using this stored fat, human beings were able to walk for long periods of time in search of food and shelter, or simply to escape from danger (storms, predators, volcanic eruptions and such like). Nowadays, our bodies still activate this release of fats into our blood in anticipation of our muscles carrying out work that they no longer have to do. The dangers for us are in fact quite different: if our boss gets annoyed with us, we are not going start fighting him (just as our money worries don't make us rob a bank). We simply feel stressed. As a result, the fatty acids accumulating in our blood do not get used and they end up being deposited on our arterial walls, leading to arteriosclerosis. As a consequence, what was once an advantage at the start of evolution, when food shortages were more common, today does us harm. Our diet based on industrially manufactured biscuits, cakes and pastries, fast food and sugary drinks, our social life revolving around the consumption of far too much food and alcohol, as well as our sedentary lifestyle, all give rise to metabolic changes that result in cardiovascular problems or cancers, through chronic and harmful hyperinsulinism.

Nowadays we are suffering from the murky side of this situation: once there were no supermarkets, processed products, bakeries and chocolate eggs with a surprise hidden inside. A person who had some food tried to make maximum use of the little energy it contained. What was once of benefit to us is today killing us, because the sugar that we eat activates insulin which is making our bodies store away large quantities of fat. Since in the developed world we are no longer threatened by famine and rarely undertake any intense physical activity, these surplus calories do not get used up. In the end, we are all likely to get fat, suffer from high blood pressure, diabetes and arthrosis, not to mention the risk of heart attacks.

To sum up, it could be said that our original primitive physiology, which remains absolutely unchanged today, was designed for a ketogenic diet (of the Dukan type or equivalent). We are made to eat a diet of fish, herbs and spices, meat, vegetables: high fibre, very low carbohydrate. We may also eat some fruit but in small quantities, since it contains fast-release sugar (most fruit is therefore harmful to our health). For evolutionary reasons as well as common sense, the Dukan Diet is not at odds with our physiology: it does not damage our health, contrary to what is claimed by certain 'experts', who of course may have their own interests at stake.

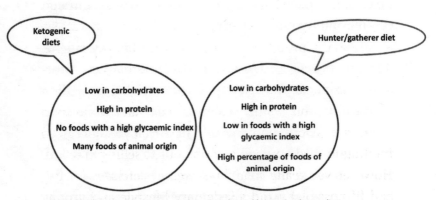

Similarities between ketogenic diets and traditional hunter/gatherer diets.

As you can see (and as has been proved by Dr Loren Cordain's team from the University of Colorado), our ancestors, who have passed on their genes to us, ate a diet that is very similar to the ketogenic diet. Conversely, it has been proved that diets with a high level of carbohydrates, and in particular those based around foods with a high glycaemic index (a criterion used to classify foods containing carbohydrates: the higher the glycaemic index, the more suddenly the food sends 'sugar' into the blood, bringing about rapid production of fats), are linked to complaints such as metabolic syndrome, Alzheimer's disease, macular degeneration (age-related retinal disease), cataracts and cancer.

3. Does this diet really work, or is it a con? [16, 17]

YES, IT IS VERY EFFECTIVE! As was explained in the answer to the previous question, this is the diet our ancestors ate and which has been passed down to us genetically; not only do we lose weight with this diet but we also avoid getting present-day illnesses (high blood pressure, diabetes, cancer, arthritis, hypercholesterolaemia, heart attacks and so on.)

In stating this, I don't mean that you have to resort to wearing loincloths and animal furs or that you have to go hunting to feed yourself or think about selling your car. However, you really should take some exercise every day and (if possible) avoid a sedentary lifestyle and driving everywhere. So go for short walks (with your partner or with friends, it is really nice and relaxing), cut down on sugar, drink plenty of water, eat fibre and more herbs and spices and vegetables rather than certain fruits. You'll see how much better you feel, that your weight will be more satisfactory and your health will improve. Fantastic! All this advice is the Dukan Diet's advice. Finally, another argument in support of this diet is the success it has had with the people best placed to judge its results – namely, those who actually use it.

4. Why does it work? [16–20]

This diet works for three main reasons:

1. Since carbohydrate intake is reduced, insulin is only slightly activated. Consequently, fat does not get stored away in the body. What is more, at the same time, insulin antagonistic hormones – the growth hormone glucagon, glucocorticoids and catecholamines – becomes activated; this enables improved insulin resistance and better use can be made of the fats, so that normal bodily functions (including glycaemia) can be maintained while at the same time ensuring considerable advantages for the body.

2. Because proteins produce a greater thermogenic effect than fats and sugar. What is thermogenesis? Induced by food, it is the amount of energy used to digest and metabolize the food we eat. If, for

example, we consume 2,000 calories a day, about 150–200 calories will be used directly (and therefore lost) as we chew, digest and store these foods. When we eat a lot of protein, the thermogenesis is greater than if we eat fat or sugar; by eating fish and meat, we use up more energy so there is less left to store away as fat.

3. As a nutrient, nitrogen is found only in proteins, so when we eat enough of them, the body's nitrogen balance is maintained. As a result, our muscles are also maintained. Weight is lost by burning up our own body fat, without us becoming malnourished or losing muscle mass.

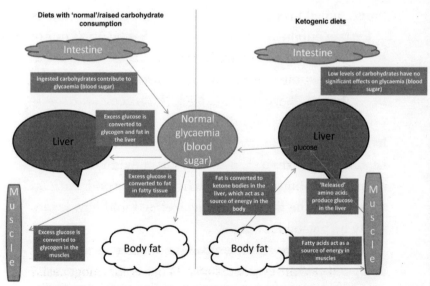

Metabolic differences between diets with a normal/raised intake of carbohydrates and ketogenic diets. (*Adapted from the Manual de Patología General* (*Manual of General Pathology*) by S. Castro del pozo)

As the diagram shows, ketogenic diets keep glycaemia at a normal level. We'll see later on that they are not dangerous for diabetics. Furthermore, using up stored fat for fuel reduces the harmful accumulation of fats and avoids excessive blood glucose levels, which poses a real danger (arteriosclerosis, infections, cancer, etc.) to health.

5. Are there any side effects? [16, 17]

NO! As we'll see throughout this book, many studies show that high-protein diets, like Dukan, have no side effects if they are followed properly. Quite the reverse, they offer many beneficial effects for our health. Remember that these diets are what we are genetically programmed to eat.

Certain opponents of the ketogenic diet refer to Professor Grande Covián, one of Spain's most renowned nutritionists, attributing to him criticism that he has never voiced. If we read his book, *Nutrition and Health. Myths, dangers and mistakes in diets*, we note that he criticizes the Atkins diet for imposing no restriction on lipids, i.e. fats: he makes a clear distinction between the Atkins diet and the Dukan Diet, which he does not condemn. On the contrary, he lists its beneficial effects and how it can really help you lose weight.

Once more, we see that criticism often lacks relevance and good faith. Never trust anyone who uses the principle of authority as an argument.

6. What is the yo-yo effect? [21-23]

The yo-yo effect is when you put back on all the weight you've lost and more, so that you end up weighing more than you did previously. The general public is fond of dwelling on this aspect of dieting. In actual fact, scientifically informed nutritionists know that the yo-yo effect as such does not exist.

After a diet, there are in reality two situations: either the dieter has learnt a lesson from the diet and has managed to alter, if only slightly, the habits that made them put on weight: if they do put the pounds back on, it will only be a partial regain; or they have learnt nothing and the lost pounds go back on again.

When you start a diet, you eat what it prescribes. If you follow the instructions properly, you lose weight; how quickly depends on what foods are used. However, it all comes down to what happens afterwards. Almost always, diets finish off with some common-sense recommendations about moderation and a balanced diet – 'you must eat when you are hungry and stop eating when you aren't any longer', this sort of thing. With such vague guidance and so little structure, very few people succeed in stabilizing their weight. They start putting weight back on. However, the pounds regained at this time are so deceptive that this weight regain takes place amid disarray, unchecked and without moderation. In fact it is thought that after dieting, in the first year weight regain is 80 per cent and 96 per cent by the end of the third year. Yet we cannot talk about a yo-yo effect. For anyone following a badly designed diet with vague recommendations it has more to do with a *rebound effect*: the body puts back on the pounds it has shed, then it stabilizes at its normal level.

Some people believe that after dieting the body's metabolism changes: the body has reacted to the diet, with the result that the pounds regained are greater than before. This is not what happens. In reality, studies prove that your metabolism stays the same. After a rebound effect that rides on top of the weight regain, metabolism returns to its initial level.

It is very easy to put weight back on. After you've finished dieting, to put on around a stone in one year all you need to do is eat an extra 80–120 calories per day! And among all that you eat every day – one full-milk yoghurt, a small croissant, three or four cups of coffee with sugar, an additional slice of pizza, a few extra chips – these surplus calories are hardly visible. Which is why it is so easy to see how people can creep back up to their initial weight and even add some more if they have not really taken the diet on board and/or if they are going though stressful or difficult times.

What is good about the Dukan Diet is that the 'after' is really thought through. The Consolidation then the Stabilization phases, plus being obliged to stick to three principles for the rest of your days, all firmly embeds what has been taught and learnt during the diet's Attack and Cruise phases.

As you can see from the table below, an individual's long-term metabolism does not change. So, then, let's stop talking about yo-yo effects and instead focus the spotlight on our laziness. With willpower, it is always possible to lose weight.

	Rodents	Primates
Glucose when fasting	decreases	decreases
Insulin when fasting	decreases	decreases
Sensitivity to insulin	increases	increases
Energy expenditure (long term)	**no difference**	**no difference**
Energy expenditure (short term)	decreases	decreases
Inflammatory mediators	decrease	decrease

The benefits of calorie restriction in rodents and higher primates.

7. Is there a yo-yo effect with the Dukan Diet?[21–23]

We have seen that the yo-yo effect does not exist – so it doesn't exist for the Dukan Diet either! What is more, if the Dukan method is followed to the letter, with a little determination and encouragement, and by following the tips and advice suggested, you won't slide back to your initial weight and you will get to an ideal weight while remaining in good health. In other words, the Dukan method is one of those rare diets offering a rule of life that can keep us at the right weight, without too much effort and under 'realistic' conditions; as Dukan says, we can enjoy 'two celebration meals' a week without this having any repercussions on our weight. For our security, we just need to stick to 'protein Thursdays', a daily 20-minute walk and no lifts or escalators, as well as the three tablespoons of oat bran.

8. Is the Dukan Diet healthy or harmful, or does it have no impact at all on health? [17, 24–30]

First of all, long-term use of ketogenic diets shows that such diets are beneficial for our health. Moreover, diets like Dukan are similar to that used daily by our ancestors, and remember that we still have the same physiology and the same nutritional needs as the first humans who survived through adverse conditions. This phylogenetic argument is of great significance. Today, palaeontologists are working to describe objectively and scientifically how our ancestors fed themselves for 190,000 years. Careful, attentive examination of their remains, of pollen, abandoned bones and grain scattered over the ground shows beyond doubt that prehistoric man (the 'universal hunter-gatherer') lived in part from hunting and fishing as well as from what he could scavenge: leaves, wild grasses (forerunners of today's seasonal cereals), berries (equivalent to our red fruits) and so on. Prehistoric man fed himself more or less on proteins and wild vegetables as well as on a few rare sources of carbohydrates that were packed with fibre but with little sugar. Our bodies are designed and programmed to eat this way – combined with a dose of physical activity we civilized humans can scarcely imagine! In fact, it is not this type of food that is harmful or dangerous but everything that has been added to it in the past 60 years; and most especially carbohydrates because although we have less and less need of them they are in abundance all around us.

Finally, lots of studies have been published proving that for the treatment of epilepsy, diabetes, obesity, arteriosclerosis, Alzheimer's disease, metabolic syndrome and cancer, a ketogenic diet has beneficial effects. We'll come back to this later.

9. Can I follow this diet, If I am diabetic? [17, 31–45]

Yes, absolutely! Today there are many studies that prove that the Dukan type of ketogenic diet does not harm the health of diabetic patients. On the contrary, this kind of diet always improves their health and also their lipid profile (cholesterol and triglyceride levels in the blood), just as it helps to better control glycaemia.

Those people with the most to gain from a ketogenic diet are diabetic and obese patients. Lots of studies have compared this diet with both the Mediterranean diet and the one advocated by the American Diabetes Association. The results prove that of all three diets the only one that improves the patient's lipid profile is the ketogenic diet. In other words, diabetics following this diet saw the good cholesterol (HDL) levels in their blood go up and their triglycerides go down. In addition, the ketogenic diet is the one that helps you lose the most weight (4–7lb /2–4kg more than the other diets, on average). It is much better at controlling glycaemia than the other two: the glycated haemoglobin level (a biological value that determines glucose concentration in the blood over three months), a crucial parameter in diabetes control, drops by 2 percentage points.

Patients with 'pre-diabetes' ('intolerance to carbohydrates' according to medical literature) benefit enormously from diets like Dukan (low in carbohydrates and lipids). As nutritionist Dr Kelly Meckling's Canadian team has proved, the diets that most improve insulin resistance are low-carbohydrate diets. If recommended at a very early stage and if enough weight is lost, with these diets it is possible to put a stop to the process of becoming diabetic. By sticking to these good habits over the long term, pre-diabetic patients will avoid getting diabetes. If we adopt eating habits such as those suggested in the Dukan Diet, our cardiovascular risk factors and chronic illnesses decrease through a reduction in blood pressure levels and in the fat and sugar in our blood, while at the same time an improved insulin response is encouraged.

In patients following a Dukan type of ketogenic diet, the weight loss observed comes about because fat stores get used up, not protein in the muscles, or because the body loses its water, as some critics would have us believe without basing this on any scientific facts whatsoever.

Many nutritionists who oppose the Dukan Diet

maintain that diabetics should not follow a ketogenic diet but should instead eat a 'normal' diet of foods with a low glycaemic index; in other words, foods that do not bring about a sharp increase in blood sugar levels. If these doctors and nutritionists had read and studied the research from the past 10 years in this area, they would have reached the following conclusions:

1. Clinical trials have proved that Dukan-type diets offer better dietary management for diabetes, than low glycaemic index diets, because a far greater weight loss can be achieved as well as better insulin control for the body.
2. In the medium term, it has been observed that twice as many patients following a Dukan type of ketogenic diet manage to reduce their medication or give it up for good than those on a non-ketogenic diet (based on low glycaemic index foods).

Likewise, Dr Farres's team from the Institute for Biomedical Research in Catalonia has recently begun to establish a molecular connection between type 2 diabetes and the beneficial metabolic changes that take place in the body with a ketogenic diet. This sort of research is paving the way for a wide range of possible treatments for diabetes, as well as for cardiovascular diseases and Alzheimer's disease.

If you are diabetic, I imagine your endocrinologist or diabetologist will have advised you to strictly control your glycaemia so as to delay the onset of complications such as renal damage (diabetic nephropathy). Indeed, once this is full-blown there is no way of reversing it; to hold back further renal damage all you can do is manage your weight, take regular exercise and continue taking medication to prevent even further damage. However, things may well change . . . As it happens, a research group from Yale University and the Mount Sinai Medical Center in New York has recently published a very interesting study that offers hope of ketogenic diets being able to repair the kidney damage caused by diabetes. Even if it is too soon to arrive at any definite conclusions, this is a first step towards understanding the physiopathology of renal damage in diabetics. This advance will help us be more open to paradigm changes in the field of medicine. Tomorrow, renal lesions caused by diabetes might well be repairable.

Proven benefits of ketogenic diets in diabetic patients
A decrease in insulin resistance
A decrease in glycated haemoglobin (HbA1c)
Lower blood pressure
Improved lipid profile (essentially due to the increase in good cholesterol)
A reduced risk of cardiovascular problems
Reversibility of diabetic nephropathy?

In conclusion, I would like to underline the following fact. Opponents of the Dukan Diet often state that the diet is dangerous for diabetics as it may bring about 'diabetic acidoketosis' (the medical consequence of over-production of ketone bodies, used by the body as an energy source when there is no glucose) with symptoms of hyperglycaemia and ketonaemia (when ketone bodies are found in the blood) in conjunction with abdominal pains. But as we have seen above, this is totally incorrect. And, in fact, the very opposite is true, since the Dukan Diet helps control diabetes and actually prevents the onset of this complication.

To sum up, the Dukan Diet helps diabetics to reduce medication (and quite often even to manage to give it up altogether). It improves parameters for cardiovascular risk without causing diabetic acidoketosis. Lastly, it might even reduce or reverse diabetic nephropathy.

10. Is it true that athletes should not follow the Dukan Diet because it makes you lose muscle mass? [17, 18, 46–48]

This statement is one of the myths and untruths doing the rounds about this type of diet, even among doctors with a special interest in nutrition and metabolism! The Dukan Diet and other ketogenic diets are particularly recommended for overweight athletes for the simple reason that they are packed with proteins of a high nutritional value and get you to lose weight by attacking your fat without touching either muscles or water. Athletes preparing for competitions use powdered proteins, as do people seeking to strengthen and develop their muscle structure.

For normal weight athletes, this diet seems to produce beneficial effects in that they have greater resistance for aerobic sports (such as running, gymnastics and cycling). Likewise, anyone, athlete or not, can follow this diet, at least during the maintenance phase (with the famous protein-only day that gets the body to cleanse itself of all the past week's excesses after partying, drinking and eating unwisely).

11. I've been told that you could become undernourished following this diet – is this true? [17–19]

This is totally untrue. As many studies from the past decade have shown, weight loss when on the diet is not connected to water or muscle mass depletion but to the loss of adipose tissue which becomes the main source of fuel for the body. This makes our fat rolls disappear – just as the risk of diabetes or cardiac arrest disappears too! Furthermore, it is not true that the diet causes osteoporosis, nor that it damages the liver and kidneys.

Even if we were fasting and drinking only water, it would take over a month before we started to become undernourished. At this point we would derive sustenance from the proteins in our muscles – but only once all the body's fat reserves have been used up. Each day, our bodies naturally burn up 20–30 grams of protein; to avoid negative protein levels, we have to eat at least 20–30 grams of protein a day to keep stable. And given that the Dukan Diet allows free access to proteins, we don't need to worry about becoming undernourished. Nor do we have to worry about not getting enough vitamins and minerals; the animal proteins allowed in the Dukan Diet contain 12 of the 13 vitamins vital for the body, as well as all the right minerals. As for number 13 – vitamin C! – it is naturally present of course in the vegetables that we eat as soon as the diet's second phase begins.

12. Is there any risk of kidney stones?[17, 49–54]

In an important article by Dr. Joaquín Pérez-Guisado of the University of Córdoba, *Ketogenic diets: additional benefits to weight loss and unfounded secondary effects*, we learn that ketogenic diets do not alter renal function and do not produce kidney stones. The beneficial effect of these diets on the kidneys is such that it has been proved (on rats) that they are capable of reversing the course of end-stage renal lesions caused by diabetes.

The unfounded rumour about kidney stones goes back to the start of the twentieth century. At that time it was said that if you were on a diet you should not drink too much water, because this could stop the production of ketone bodies and their positive effects. However, we have known for a long time now that taking in liquids does not lessen the beneficial effects of the diet. In fact, we are advised to keep well hydrated as this is vital for getting rid of waste products, and dilating the stomach in a purely mechanical way makes us feel full.

The average prevalence of renal lithiasis (stones) in the general population of industrialized countries across the world is between 5 and 10 per cent. The prevalence of kidney stones in people following a traditional (i.e. low-calorie) diet is around 5 per cent – and it is absolutely the same for patients on ketogenic diets. So what do these results tell us? First of all, they prove that people on the diet are less likely to develop kidney stones. Kidney stones occur primarily when a person does not drink enough. Studies in the United States have shown that over half the adult population is chronically dehydrated and has lost the physiological signals for thirst, with dehydration resulting first and foremost in a desire to eat.

Let's summarize: by following the Dukan Diet's first recommendation, which is to drink 2 litres of water a day, you run *no risk whatsoever* of developing a kidney stone. On the other hand, if you are not on this diet or if you are following any other diet and drinking only a little water, it is possible that you will develop stones (especially if your body is susceptible to creating kidney stones).

13. Is this an unnatural diet? [15, 17]

Not only is it not unnatural, but it is also the diet that comes closest to what our ancestors ate; let's remind ourselves that we still have the same physiology and the same genes as prehistoric man. Consequently, the closer we get to eating the food that allowed him to survive adverse geographical and nutritional conditions, the more 'natural' our food will be. We will feel better physically, we will suffer less illness and we will be able to grow old slowly, while enjoying a better quality of life.

In the 1980s, the Food and Agriculture Organization (FAO) of the United Nations laid out its recommendations for a 'natural' balanced diet: 55–60 per cent carbohydrates, 15–20 per cent proteins and 20–25 per cent fats. And yet, following on from these recommendations, there has been a spectacular rise in obesity in all age groups, as there has been in type 2 diabetes, cardiovascular problems and cancer. Moreover, these recommendations have never been proved to be appropriate and healthy.

Conversely, these are many studies that point to how ketogenic diets are more therapeutic and help to prevent the great curses of the twenty-first century: obesity, heart attacks, diabetes, arthrosis and metabolic syndrome. So if we rely on our good old common sense, we note that the Dukan Diet, in its first two purely weight-loss phases, is very similar to our ancestors' diet – the diet for which our bodies have been programmed and which absolutely suits us down to the ground. However, the recommendations from the FAO and nutritionists have become a dogma that is creating health problems. So then, of the two which is the most 'natural' diet? The ketogenic diet, of course.

Type of diet	Hunter-gatherer	FAO recommendations
Carbohydrates	20–40 %*	55–60 %
Proteins	20–30 %	15–20 %
Fats	20–30 %	20–25 %

A comparison between the hunter-gatherer diet and the FAO's recommendations.

As you can see from this table, the diet that we ought to follow based on our genes, our lifestyle and physiology has nothing in common with what the health and food authorities suggest we consume.

Moreover, if we compare the Dukan Diet with the LEARN (Lifestyle, Exercise, Attitude, Relationships and Nutrition) diet (55–60 per cent carbohydrates and physical exercise, as recommended by the FAO) and the Zone diet (40 per cent carbohydrates), we see that it is the Dukan Diet that offers better weight loss, better muscle protection and better effects on metabolism.

So from now on, whenever anyone tells you that the Dukan Diet is not natural, as well as not paying them any heed, encourage these people to go and look up the scientific literature using the American National Library of Medicine website (this is very easy). This way your critic will be able to read up on the subject and so stop peddling preconceived ideas.

---

*   In this diet, the carbohydrates are mostly low glycaemic index (remember that almost all fruit has a high glycaemic index).

14 . Are there any risks or drawbacks from not eating fruit during the first two phases of the Dukan Diet? [55–60]

NO! The European study on the role of nutrition in reducing cardiac risk recently published by Dr Crowe and her team in Oxford proves that the amount of fruit eaten daily does not impact on survival rates. In addition, NOT EATING FRUIT DURING THE ATTACK PHASE DOES NOT PUT US AT ANY RISK because this phase lasts only 3–7 days. As soon as we start the Cruise phase, we can eat vegetables 'as much as we want'; vegetables are healthier than most fruit, as we shall see below. With as many vitamins and mineral salts as fruit, the advantage of vegetables is that they do not contain simple sugars. So you have nothing to fear from going without fruit – vegetables are fruit without the sugar.

Here is a third reason for not worrying about there being no fruit during the diet's first two phases: high in fast (rapid-absorption) sugars, fruit contributes to the growth of cancerous cells and their development (metastases). Dr Johannes Coy, a cancer researcher at the German Cancer Research Centre in Heidelberg, believes that lemons are the only really healthy fruit that we can eat in unlimited quantities! Conversely, bananas, raisins, figs and dried apricots should be avoided as they are a factor in helping cancers develop and spread. In other words, if you have a cancer and eat large amounts of high-sugar fruit, this cancer is likely to spread more quickly than if you were following a low-carbohydrate (or no-carbohy-drate) diet. You may even be able to limit your cancer from developing with a no-carbs diet.

Lastly, as Dr Bharat Aggarwal from the Anderson Cancer Center in Houston (where celebrities go for cancer treatment) says in his excellent book, *Healing Spices*: 'By including only vegetables and fruit in your diet, you will not win the battle against this disease as the real secret to ward it off and prolong your life is a diet full of SPICES!'

Yes, that is indeed what you read: turmeric, cinnamon, cardamom, black pepper and so on. Spices contain an array of unique phytochemicals, which means that they can fight the disease and sometimes cure it. The countries with a low rate of cancer, cardiovascular diseases, diabetes and obesity, such as India, Japan and China, are not those where the most fruit is consumed daily but the ones where one or several sorts of these spices are eaten every day.

The good news is that the Dukan Diet does not stop you from eating spices (in any of its phases). Quite the contrary, it encourages you to make use of them, since apart from their beneficial health effects, spices can also improve the flavour of foods and make them really tasty.

15. Does the Dukan Diet contribute to the onset of cancer? [17, 24, 57, 61–145]

Although nowadays their recommendations are out of date, the FAO and World Health Organization (WHO) continue to state that carbohydrates should comprise 45–60 per cent of our diet. Recent research proves quite the reverse, that too many carbohydrates are bad for our health as they provide the basic fuel for cancerous cells. In fact, by trying to prevent the cancer from getting carbohydrates, we have a means of controlling and even stopping it. To achieve this objective, Dr Johannes Coy (see above) suggests that daily sugar intake should not exceed 1 gram per kilo (just over 2lb) of body weight. So, for example, I weigh 79 kilos (just under 12½ stone) which means I should not eat more than 79 grams of carbohydrates per day. To make this easy to work out, in his book, *The new anti-cancer diet*, Dr Coy sets out different coloured tables. The green foods, containing few carbohydrates, can be eaten in unlimited quantities. Even if they are healthy, the yellow foods need to be monitored because, beyond a certain daily intake, blood sugar levels increase, enabling the cancer to feed itself. Finally, foods on the red list are generally not recommended as they contain too many sugars that get rapidly assimilated. What we find on this last list in particular is fruit – another reason for considering that often fruit does us more harm than good.

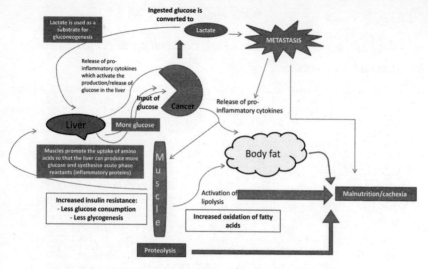

Cancer metabolism. Note that tumour cells feed solely on sugar (adapted from Klement RJ et al. *Nutrition & Metabolismo (Nutrition and Metabolism)* 2011; 8:75

In this table, we can see that metabolism in cancerous cells is fundamentally based on using up glucose and creating inflammation which results in muscle proteins and fat being destroyed so that the liver has more substrates, enabling it to produce more glucose to better feed the cancer. Consequently, we can state that not only does the Dukan Diet not cause cancer but it actually helps prevent it and even limits its development, as we shall see later on when we analyse different research papers about patients suffering from various forms of the disease.

16. Why does this diet have so many critics? [23]

There are several reasons for this, and each critic may be motivated by one or other, or even several, of them:

Because of health professionals' ignorance and lack of interest.

When ketogenic diets appeared, they were hastily condemned by the so-called 'experts' in the field. In the 1980s, the doctors and nutritionists who listened to this unfounded criticism never bothered to study and analyse the current scientific data. They simply carried on repeating the same nonsense, heard 30 years ago, that the diet would be bad for the liver and for diabetes, it would be unnatural, it would cause undernourishment, and so on. What is most striking, and most sad, is that since 2002, when the first data showing the benefits of the Atkins diet were presented at the American national cardiology conference, these professionals still have not found the time to seek more information on the subject.

Because health professionals think they know everything.

Working as doctors, we are the experts; the general public expects us to have expertise in a wide range of subjects. Since we think we've got a very good grip of physiology, we like to use our 'magical reasoning' – and there we have it! I have even seen an endocrinologist on television showing drawings of a sturdily built man losing his biceps because of the diet, which is totally untrue and proves that the 'experts' do not know as much as they think. For more information on this subject, I recommend you read my book, *What your doctor should know to save your life.*

For economic reasons.

Most of the people who criticize the Dukan Diet are dietitians and professionals who offer diets through their own private consultations. Until the Dukan Diet appeared they were earning a lot of money. Since this diet is easy to follow on your own at home or with help from the internet, it has resulted in a considerable loss of income for these practitioners. This is why they have all set about weaving a tissue of lies, in order to keep hold of clients who try to slim down every year without ever achieving successful results.

Because of the Einstein effect.

Albert Einstein said that it was easier to destroy an atom than it was to change an idea. What he meant was that human beings are more stubborn-minded than we think; it is difficult to change accepted ideas, especially if our parents have passed them on to us and if we embraced them when we were young, treating them as dogma or as the principles for our professional work. Although working as doctors, we are scientists; we still remain swayed by certain prejudices that stop us from taking new information on board if it runs counter to the ideas we already hold.

Among such prejudices, the following should be highlighted:

- *Previously held beliefs*: we tend to search and retain any information that backs up knowledge we have previously acquired and we reject anything that does not fit with what we believe. Yet some critics of the Dukan Diet have read books praising the virtues of ketogenic diets; however, since at the outset they did not believe in these diets, reading about them did nothing to change their minds. They carry on thinking that these diets are bad for our health. On the other hand, such people are more open to works that back up their convictions.

- *Social influence* and group opinion have a tendency to dominate and control the individual. If you believed in ketogenic diets 10 years ago but you were continually in contact with colleagues who looked upon them as the worst possible diet, you would end up thinking like them and also rejecting such diets. It would be the wrong choice but as the psychologist Professor Daniel T. Gilbert of Harvard University has proved in his article, 'How mental systems believe', we are not sceptical by nature: not to believe in a very widely held (but false) theory requires great mental effort. It is easy to fall in with group opinion.

- *Receptivity*: the most recent information is the information we use most frequently. Since we constantly hear that a balanced diet should be made up of 60 per cent carbohydrates, 15 per cent proteins and 25 per cent fats (even though, as we have said, this macronutrient breakdown is unhealthy), when we compare this breakdown to the Dukan Diet or any other ketogenic diet, we tell ourselves that such diets are bound to be unhealthy as they diverge too greatly from official recommendations – yet another mistake that emanates from our system of reasoning.

As has been proved many times, in medicine it takes about 50 years for knowledge to reach the doctors! So it is best not to worry – in 20 years' time, your dietitian will be prescribing the Dukan Diet and its variations.

17. When I'm losing weight, is it fat that I'm going to lose – and not muscle or water?[17, 146, 147]

Some of those who criticize the Dukan method say that weight loss is fast because you also lose muscle and water. Here again, we have people without all the information. Why would you lose your muscle by eating animal meat, the muscle from fish, chicken and beef?

Many studies on patients have shown that weight is lost primarily from the body's fat supplies. Among these studies, attention should be drawn to the one carried out by the University of Kansas School of Medicine: after diabetic and obese patients had followed a ketogenic diet for 16 weeks, an average weight loss of just over 1½ stone (around 10 kilos) was recorded through a reduction of approximately 10 per cent of body fat.

After analysing the effects of Dukan-type high-protein diets, the eminent Spanish nutritionist Francisco Grande

Covián reached the conclusion that weight loss is proportionate to the length of treatment; this loss occurring mainly at the expense of body fat.

In other studies carried out on overweight or obese people it has been proved that a regime of endurance and bodybuilding exercises combined with a low-carb diet causes body fat to disappear without any loss of muscle mass. The other way round, using a traditional, non-ketogenic diet that is not low-carb may increase muscle mass but less body fat is shed. As a result, the desired positive effects – i.e. loss of excess body fat – are much reduced with conventional diets.

As for eliminating water, studies prove that as such this does not exist. For the first days of the diet, you will need to urinate frequently because of ketogenesis and this will be evident; however, this is very quickly counterbalanced by the amount of water you drink daily. After a week, the initial effect will no longer have any impact and any weight loss you record will be due only to fat loss.

18. Will I lose muscle mass? [17–19, 46–48, 146, 147]

We mentioned this above but we'll go over it again and explain it in greater detail. You will not lose muscle mass! There are several reasons for this:

- Within our bodies are two processes that coexist: one is building the body daily and the other is breaking it down. To maintain our internal equilibrium and structure, we eliminate 20–30 grams of protein a day as amino acids (the building blocks of proteins). If the body gets these 20–30 grams replenished through food, our protein level remains balanced and there is no need for the body to draw on its muscle mass. Since protein intake with the Dukan Diet is more than ample, there is no need to worry about your muscles; there is no loss of muscle. Moreover, many studies prove that this type of diet can improve athletes' performance, especially during aerobic exercises – further evidence that there is no muscle loss.

- Once your carbohydrate stores have been used up, the body turns to its fat stores to find energy. It is only once these fat stores have been exhausted (after about 3–4 weeks of fasting) that the body starts plundering its muscles. Therefore, as the Dukan Diet sets no restrictions regarding quantities for the foods you are allowed, and since many of these are high-protein foods, you don't need to fear for your biceps.

- What is more, the proteins in your muscles are so important and so invaluable to the body that, even in the worst circumstances of food shortage, resources get activated so that your muscles and their proteins are protected.

On this most important point, I will conclude by reiterating that you would need to *go for three weeks without eating* before you began to lose any muscle mass. With the high-protein Dukan Diet which allows copious quantities – and which contractually compels you to walk every day and give up taking lifts and escalators – not only will you not lose any muscle, but, quite the opposite, you will in fact gain muscle! You will look slimmer even though you may weigh the same, because muscle takes up less space than fat.

19. Does this diet provide enough calcium and does it cause osteoporosis? [148–153]

When calcium is metabolized normally (sufficient calcium intake plus correct hormonal activity) and combined with adequate daily physical exercise (walking, for example, for 30 minutes) this wards off and prevents osteoporosis. In the Dukan Diet, calcium intake is not reduced. However, since you can also drink skimmed milk and eat 0% fat yoghurt every day, throughout all four phases, there is no scientific reason at all why you should suffer from osteoporosis.

As Dr Pérez-Guisado has shown, the osteoporosis that is supposedly caused by ketogenic diets is just an idea hawked around by certain malicious critics who are not scientists. It is a side effect that simply does not exist.

20. Are there any studies comparing the effectiveness of this diet with other diets?[154–169]

A great number of studies compare ketogenic diets with other diets. The main ones compared are:

- the American Diabetes Association diet
- the standard Mediterranean diet
- the GI diet (based on low glycaemic index foods)
- the low-fat and high-carb diet
- hypolipidemic diets
- the LEARN diet (55–60 per cent carbohydrates and physical exercise etc.)
- the Ornish diet (vegetarian)
- the Zone diet (or the 'happy medium' diet)
- a traditional diet, for children with severe epilepsy that is difficult to control pharmacologically

21. According to these comparative studies which is the best diet? [17, 154–169]

From all these comparisons, it has been proved that the ketogenic diet is both the most effective and the healthiest, because it helps:

- improve the blood lipid profile
- better control diabetes

- produce greater weight loss, taken from body fat
- reduce cardiovascular risks
- prevent cancer
- improve treatment for cancer patients
- lower blood pressure
- reduce insulin resistance
- better control epilepsy in children
- improve athletes' physical performance

By following the Dukan Diet, you will be able to attain your ideal weight and improve your health. The concrete and not-too-frustrating stabilization programme that the Dukan Diet offers will not expose you to any risks from possible side effects; on the contrary, you stand to gain much from it.

22. Can I eat eggs on protein-only days? [57,170]

It has long been known that eggs are highly nutritious. Yet many doctors advise against eating lots of eggs, believing that the yolks increase blood cholesterol levels, which is a truth that has become firmly rooted in the collective subconscious.

The experts ought to be well aware that in reality there are two types of cholesterol – exogenous (obtained from the food we eat) and endogenous (made by the liver, even if you don't eat any food containing cholesterol). It has been proven that what is obtained from outside the body (exogenous) has only a very minor impact on blood cholesterol levels.

57

What is more, a recent study has shown that eating up to six eggs a day (!) meant it was possible to cut down the risk factors associated with metabolic syndrome. Finally, eggs appear on Dr Johannes Coy's green list of foods (see also question 15) that can be eaten every day, without restriction, because they protect us from cancer.

Armed with all these arguments, don't think twice about eating an egg a day, during all the Dukan Diet phases (including the protein-only days).

23. If I eat eggs regularly, will this increase my cholesterol level? [57, 170]

Recent studies compared two groups of obese patients who had been on a Dukan-style diet. The first group ate six eggs a day, the second followed the diet but without eating any eggs. Weight loss was as expected in both groups, and in each group the patients had the same results with regard to the drop in lipid levels in the blood. However, the group on six eggs a day saw a significant increase in good cholesterol (HDL) and at the same time their cardiovascular risk factors also dropped (triglyceride levels, the percentage of body fat and blood pressure all decreased).

Changes after 12 weeks on a low-carbohydrate diet	
% fat	
group 1 (6 eggs/day)	-5.4%
group 2 (0 eggs/day)	-6.1%
*Systolic blood pressure**	
group 1 (6 eggs/day)	-0.5mmHg
group 2 (0 eggs/day)	-0.1mmHg
Diastolic blood pressure	
group 1 (6 eggs/day)	-10.6mmHg
group 2 (0 eggs/day)	-4.6mmHg
Total cholesterol	
group 1 (6 eggs/day)	+3.9mg/dl
group 2 (0 eggs/day)	+1.0mg/dl
'Good' cholesterol – HDL	
group 1 (6 eggs/day)	+12mg/dl
group 2 (0 eggs/day)	-1.2mg/dl
'Bad' cholesterol – LDL	
group 1 (6 eggs/day)	+16.8mg/dl
group 2 (0 eggs/day)	+13.5mg/dl
Triglycerides	
group 1 (6 eggs/day)	-44.1mg/dl
group 2 (0 eggs/day)	-49.4mg/dl

The changes in cholesterol, triglyceride levels in the blood, blood pressure and the percentage of body fat in obese patients after following a low-carb diet for 12 weeks (group 1: 6 eggs a day; group 2: not allowed to eat any eggs at all).

---

* *The higher blood pressure reading: for example, 120 if the blood pressure reading is 120/80. No significant differences were found between the group eating eggs and the one not eating eggs.*

As you can see from this table, eating eggs in conjunction with the ketogenic diet results in a considerable increase in good cholesterol, an average drop of 10mmHg in blood pressure and triglyceride levels in the blood dropped by over 40mg/dl. This means that by eating eggs, not only is there no significant increase in bad cholesterol but you can also improve your good cholesterol level and curb the risk of heart attacks and cardiovascular problems.

24. Can children and teenagers follow the Dukan Diet?[17]

Yes! The Dukan Diet is not contraindicated whatsoever for children or teenagers, especially if they are carrying extra pounds or are obese. Dr Dukan does not suggest that children use his diet because they would require specific supervision. However, it has been seen that this diet could be enormously useful for children and teenagers suffering with severe epilepsy that does not respond to medication. Moreover, different studies of such young people put on a carbohydrate-free diet have not shown any side effects at all.

As a precautionary measure, it is advisable to ensure that children following a Dukan (or ketogenic) diet remain well hydrated because they tend to drink less and become dehydrated, which could result in kidney stones. A tip for an easy way to make sure that children stay hydrated is simply to buy the sugar-free, zero-calorie lemonade or orangeade-type drinks readily available in supermarkets.

25. How can this diet help treat epilepsy effectively?[17, 171–187]

Already back in 1921, researchers at the Rochester Mayo Clinic in the USA had demonstrated that a Dukan-style ketogenic diet ensured that epilepsy that was unresponsive to medication could be properly controlled.

Today, there are hundreds of articles, conference and clinical trial reports that prove that this sort of diet works when treating and controlling the worst cases of epilepsy. The sheer number of cases that have been observed, including patients who had no need whatsoever to lose weight, bear witness to the fact that this diet, which has been passed on through generations of humans, is completely harmless. That there are no side effects confirms this.

All the medication used to treat serious cases of epilepsy have considerable side effects, whereas the Dukan Diet, on the other hand, is inexpensive, it works, and may prove to be an ideal, danger-free additional treatment.

26. Is the Dukan Diet also suitable for children with epilepsy?[17, 171–187]

Yes! That the ketogenic diet was suitable for all age groups was confirmed with the first studies carried out in the 1920s. According to some studies, 15 per cent of children with virtually incurable epilepsy who tried this diet over the course of a year stopped suffering attacks; 30 per cent of them experienced a 90 per cent drop in the number of attacks. Unfortunately, for the remaining 55 per cent, the diet did not work. Therefore, if for any reason the child does not tolerate the diet, or if it does not produce any significant results, the diet should be stopped.

Studies that have compared the Dukan-style ketogenic diet with the new anti-epileptic drugs have proved that the diet works, even with cases where the drugs had no effect. Which is why we advise you to consider this type of diet for children with this condition (obviously they must be supervised by experts who are completely knowledgeable about this pathology).

There are advantages in using this type of diet as a treatment. The ones to emphasize are the absence of serious, irreversible side effects, and the fact that the diet can be followed without admission to hospital (through medical supervision at home or out-patient appointments at the hospital), as researchers in America and Canada have shown. The effectiveness of the ketogenic diet does not depend on the type of epilepsy or number of attacks. It has even been observed that the diet works for certain syndromes that do not respond to medication, such as: 1) Dravet syndrome (severe epilepsy in children), 2) myoclonic epilepsy in Asia (severe epilepsy in children), 3) Rett syndrome (a genetic disorder resulting in serious disruption to the development of the central nervous system), 4) neuronal migration disorders (neurological conditions caused by a defect during the brain's development), 5) tuberous sclerosis complex (a genetic disease that results in multiple benign tumours, a major cause of epileptic attacks), and 6) De Vivo disease (a rare genetic disease that causes disruption to the brain's metabolism, characterized in particular by epileptic attacks).

It is not known whether the Dukan Diet works in synergy with anti-epileptic drugs. However, it has been shown that the diet can be rendered more effective if combined with other anti-epileptic treatments such as vagus nerve stimulation.

27. Can the diet be adapted or improved for children with epilepsy?[184, 178]

So that children find the foods a little tastier, you can slightly increase the amount of sugar and fat they eat so that following the diet will be easier. Based on published studies, we recommend starting off by sticking to the diet strictly for the first three months and then gradually increasing carbohydrate intake; but without exceeding the amount after which ketogenesis stops. If the threshold of 20 grams of carbohydrates a day is exceeded, it is highly likely that the diet will become less effective in reducing the number of epileptic attacks.

Using calorie-free sweeteners and zero-calorie fizzy drinks may be helpful in treating these epileptic children. Moreover, for children with epilepsy the diet has to be set up and monitored by hospital neurological units that specifically treat epilepsy; the treatment can be delivered without hospitalization, but it needs to be tailored to each individual child's needs.

28. Are there any studies that prove that this diet is beneficial for the treatment of epilepsy?[17, 171–187]

There are many studies that prove that the Dukan type of ketogenic diet is beneficial in the treatment of epilepsy and other neurological syndromes (as a primary treatment or to treat patients for whom medication does not work). The results published include case series studies, clinical trials and meta-analysis (the most extensive studies that can be carried out to prove whether a treatment works).

Moreover, international guidelines recommend trying diets of this type. In 2009, international neurological organizations reached a consensus about prescribing and using ketogenic diets for this type of patient, both adults and children.

29. Is it true that the Dukan Diet disrupts liver function and causes fat to accumulate in the liver? [188–190]

Although this criticism is frequently voiced, not only is the statement untrue but the very opposite happens! The Dukan Diet lightens the liver's workload and cuts down the amount of fat accumulating in tired livers. How? By cutting out the fats and alcohol that it is the liver's job to cleanse out of the body. A liver on a ketogenic diet can take a rest.

Without liaising about their work, a group of Spanish researchers and an American research team have both proved the positive effects of ketogenic diets on fat accumulation in the liver (not due to alcohol consumption).

Steatosis is the name given to accumulation of fat in the liver; it is becoming increasingly common in young people. Cirrhosis of the liver can develop as one of the consequences of non-alcoholic steatosis (fatty liver disease). Thanks to studies undertaken by Dr Pérez-Guisado in Spain and Dr Tendler in the United States, we know that the Dukan Diet – and others of the same type – are beneficial and not dangerous for treating livers that have been extremely damaged by the disease.

To sum up, the Dukan Diet does not affect the liver; quite the reverse, since it cuts down the accumulation of fat and results in positive outcomes for the liver, including an improved lipid profile and prevention of cirrhosis.

30. Can I follow this diet, If I am morbidly obese?[17]

Yes, you can follow it. What is more, there is proof that it will be most beneficial to you. Morbid obesity is associated with cardiovascular diseases, arthrosis, high cholesterol levels, diabetes, high blood pressure, sleep apnoea syndrome, and many other problems that will improve by following the Dukan Diet and other ketogenic diets in general.

Weight loss takes place because body fat is being burnt up, so you will not feel as if you are losing muscle mass or bone mass. You will gradually become less obese; your cardiovascular risk parameters will improve as well as your ability to do some exercise and take a daily walk without getting tired.

It has been observed in studies published on obese menopausal women (with a metabolism that has really slowed down) that this sort of diet brings about weight loss, improves the heart and carbohydrate levels in the blood, as well as increasing the capacity to take the aerobic exercise that contributes to our physical and mental wellbeing and general state of health.

31. Is it a good thing to follow the diet before having surgery for morbid obesity?[191]

Between 2008 and 2010, I was one of three Spanish surgeons working on the European Obesity Academy project at the Karolinska Institute in Stockholm. For this project, different clinical trials were carried out on patients with morbid obesity. The study conducted by my group was as follows: we wanted to see if a ketogenic diet followed for a fortnight before undergoing surgery for morbid obesity – which might be gastric band surgery, gastroplasty (to reduce the volume of the stomach) or a gastric bypass – would lessen complications and the amount of time required to perform the operation. The results show that the patients who do the diet lose 9–11lb (4–5kg) before the operation. Losing this weight correlates with a considerable improvement in their physiological parameters and a much reduced risk from the surgery. So I advise all patients about to undergo this sort of treatment to do the diet a few weeks before their operation.

32. Can I do the diet after the operation?

You can do the diet before or after being operated on. For the first few months after the operation, patients are recommended to follow the diet in consultation with the bariatric surgery monitoring unit in their hospital. After that, it can be followed without supervision; it will make you lose weight. Then, once you are no longer obese, you will do the diet once a week as Dr Dukan recommends. This will ensure that you do not put back on the weight you have lost and that you benefit from all the positive effects your body will enjoy (already mentioned throughout the book).

In addition, given that the average waiting time for bariatric surgery is about one year, you could start the diet while you are waiting. If you are strict and follow the instructions correctly, it is possible that you may no longer need the operation at all! Because as the date for the operation gets nearer, you will no longer be morbidly obese, or have high blood pressure and serious diabetes or the co-morbidities associated with them, which was the reason why you were meant to have the surgery. This way you will avoid a procedure that has risks and makes changes to your digestive tract – and we do not really yet know what the long-term outcomes are for this type of operation.

You will lose nothing by doing this diet! Even if you don't succeed then you can still have the operation.

33. How can I get the most out of the protein-only days?

If you have eaten and drunk a lot the day before it will be difficult for you to really benefit much from your protein day. It won't be of great use to you as your body will be full of sugars and it will take a long time to use them up. This means that by the end of your protein day it will be as if you had only done half a protein day, or even less. So here is a very simple tip. On the afternoon before your protein day, only eat the foods you are allowed. This way, you will start getting rid of all the sugar on the day before your protein day. On the following day, from the morning onwards your body will begin to draw upon its fat stores. And without putting in much effort, you will achieve far better results.

34. Will the diet improve my blood sugar and cholesterol levels?[17, 192–225]

Of course! As we have seen, the diet lowers bad and increases good cholesterol. It makes it easier to control diabetes, especially in diabetic patients, and it lowers blood pressure. It brings about many positive effects without impacting on the liver and kidneys, without causing osteoporosis or a loss of muscle mass. This means that if you want to lose weight in a healthy way, then the Dukan Diet is a highly recommended option. If you do not need to lose weight but have conditions such as type 2 diabetes or high blood pressure, take the trouble to give it a go and you will see the good results for yourself.

35. Can I follow this diet, If I have high blood pressure?[17, 192–225]

Numerous studies have proved that Dukan-style ketogenic diets lower blood pressure while at the same time improving other cardiovascular risk parameters, such as hyperglycaemia and high blood levels of cholesterol and triglycerides. Furthermore, by losing visceral fat – often connected with cardiovascular problems – our lipid profile and the condition of our liver will be improved.

36. I want to lower my bad cholesterol level (LDL) and increase my good cholesterol level (HDL) – can I follow the diet?[192–225]

You may follow it and you would even be advised to do so and without hesitation! Studies have provided proof that in obese patients with low levels of good cholesterol (HDL), the ketogenic diet considerably boosted HDL levels. At the same time, their bad cholesterol (LDL) levels dropped, along with their systolic blood pressure and their body fat levels.

Today a low HDL level is considered one of the most significant cardiovascular risk factors there is. In other words, the higher your HDL, the less risk you run of getting cardiovascular disease. Greenland Eskimos have a low incidence of heart attacks; at any rate, far fewer than the rest of the Danish population, where HDL levels are lower.

37. I have a child who is obese – can he or she do this diet?[17, 192–225]

Given that in recent years there has been an explosion in childhood obesity rates, and 7 out of 10 children are overweight and will continue to be so during adolescence and adulthood, it seems to me important to begin dealing with this problem very early on. Even with exercise and better lifestyle habits, some obese children are still unable to lose weight. To my mind, the Dukan Diet is therefore entirely appropriate.

Among the precautions to be observed, it is recommended that you supervise how much water is drunk since children can more easily become dehydrated if they fail to take in large enough quantities of liquid. If your child refuses to drink water, you can substitute a zero-calorie fizzy drink.

Remember that science already has a wide experience of using this type of diet with epileptic children and we know that these diets do not cause any significant side effects.

38. Can the Dukan Diet help fight against cancer?[17, 24, 57, 61–145]

Cancer specialists have known for a long time that metabolism in tumour cells relies almost exclusively on glucose. Consequently, if our blood sugar level is high (or even if it is not high but our daily carbohydrate intake is excessive), this may encourage tumour cells to develop and to be able to metastasize. This means that ketogenic diets have a huge role to play in treating malignant tumours. Let us remind ourselves that a normal cell can feed on glucose, fatty acids and ketone bodies – chemical products synthesized by the liver and used by the body as an energy source; in the ketogenic diet, when there is no glucose, the remaining foods become the main 'fuel' – whereas a cancerous cell can only feed on glucose. So by suppressing carbohydrate intake, the normal cells can continue to live without any difficulty but the cancerous cells will struggle to find the dose of glucose they require to feed their amazing capacity for expansion.

Dr Johannes Coy has recently studied what happens when tumours have restricted access to carbohydrates. In his book, *The new anti-cancer diet*, he classifies foods in three colour-coded tables (see also question 15):

- green (can be eaten without any restriction every day)
- yellow (can be eaten every day, but with certain limits)
- red (to be avoided as far as possible)

If you examine these tables, you will realize that all the foods on the green list are the ones that appear in phases 1 and 2 of the Dukan Diet (the same is true for the protein day foods).

In the light of the research data currently available, we can say that the Dukan Diet and the other ketogenic diets help fight against cancer. Furthermore, if we add enough spices to the Dukan Diet foods – and this is not forbidden; in fact, it is strongly recommended – we will fight cancer even more effectively.

39. Are there any studies about the diet and cancer patients?[61–145]

Yes, there are lots of studies! Those carried out in laboratories on animals, which have shown that restricting carbohydrates stops the growth of cancerous cells, as well as those on people.

Of the many studies available, we must draw attention to those carried out on patients with malignant brain tumours, where it has been demonstrated that these diets are helpful, safe and should be considered as an alternative cancer therapy. It has been proved that in patients with metastatic tumours, ketogenic diets, like Dukan, improve quality of life and blood parameters without producing any side effects.

Recent studies seem to conclude that these diets may be useful for preventing and treating prostate cancer. There is also some evidence that this type of diet may help patients with breast cancer, cancer of the colon, etc. However, further studies are still required to fully understand how this mechanism works.

40. Can I follow this diet for the rest of my life?[17, 226, 227]

Yes. In actual fact, the Dukan Diet is designed to be a 'lifetime project'. Its first phase is short but spectacular as weight loss is very fast. The second phase then takes over and allows you to lose around a couple of pounds a week. Next, once you have got down to your True Weight, the Consolidation phase builds a bridge between the actual weight-loss diet and the rest of your life (or the Stabilization phase). It is following the diet for life that makes the method a success.

It is true that, in the medium term, most diets have very high failure rates. Once dieting is over, the weight that has been lost creeps back on again, maybe with some extra pounds to boot! The Dukan Diet will be no exception to this rule if you stop once you reach your True Weight, without then continuing with the Consolidation and afterwards the lifelong Stabilization phases.

It is this aspect of the diet, not widely enough known, that makes it so unusual and innovative. Apart from the positive effects on health that we have examined, as far as I know it is the only diet that gives you a concrete, carefully planned, logical and effective programme so that you can avoid regaining the pounds you've lost.

41. Can I try this diet if I have arthritis?[228]

Recent experimental studies have proved that this type of diet can help lessen and treat the pain experienced with arthritic conditions. The ketogenic diet can help lessen inflammatory reactions, and therefore the arthritis, since one of its features is precisely this type of inflammatory process (as we saw with cancer metabolism, also caused essentially by an inflammatory process). This means that if you suffer from inflammatory arthritis, not only are there no contraindications, but following the diet could even help alleviate the symptoms. On the other hand, if you have wear-and-tear arthritis and you are obese, as well as specifically impacting your arthritis, your dieting will also reduce your weight and thereby relieve the pressure on your joints. Overall, you will see an improvement not just in your symptoms but also in your mobility, which will make for a more enriching life.

42. If I am suffering from osteoporosis and want to do this diet to lose weight, are there any contraindications? [17, 148–153]

Although all those people who criticize the Dukan Diet and other ketogenic diets never stop talking about how it leads to bone calcium loss, and therefore to osteoporosis, in reality there are no studies at all in adults following this type of diet that prove these assertions.

In children with epilepsy, loss of calcium in bones has been observed; however, there is no proof of long-term negative effects.

So from this we can conclude that if you are an adult with osteoporosis (or worried about getting it), there is no problem in following the Dukan Diet as it includes many high-calcium foods. The Dukan Diet encourages you to do sport, which in itself may also improve your symptoms, both through losing weight and by regulating calcium metabolism in your bones.

43. Can I use any form of seasoning to make my food tastier? [56, 58, 59]

Yes. In Attack, which is the phase with pure proteins and therefore the most restrictive, you may season any meal you want with herbs and spices – garlic, basil, thyme, ginger, rosemary, turmeric, pepper, cinnamon, etc. You can also do this in the other phases. As well as herbs and spices, you can use other ingredients that add flavour and texture, such as:

- onions, fresh and dried
- lemon juice
- peppers
- soy sauce, tomatoes and tomato purée
- oat bran
- vanilla
- fat-free, salt-free stock cubes
- seaweed
- aniseed
- agar-agar
- 0 per cent fat fish or meat stock

44. Can I use spices?[1–3, 56, 59]

Of course you can! As well as enhancing the flavour, spices also seem to produce a satiating effect in the brain, so they will make you feel more satisfied and nice and full without eating so much food.

And as Dr Bharat Aggarwal from the Anderson Cancer Center in Houston writes, don't forget that '*a diet full of spices helps fight diseases far more effectively and positively than diets without spices (even if these diets contain lots of fruit and vegetables)*'. So if spices are not already part of your life, then make them part of it.

Personally, in addition to my protein day and what I normally eat, every day I have a half-pot of natural yoghurt with half a teaspoonful of freshly ground black pepper and a teaspoonful of turmeric mixed in. We are going to see that many spices have the most amazing properties.

45. As well as enhancing the flavour of food, do herbs and spices have any positive effects on health?[56–59]

Since ancient times, the positive effects of herbs and spices on health have been recognized. They help to ward off chronic illnesses such as diabetes, high blood pressure, hypercholesterolaemia, Alzheimer's disease, arthritis, psoriasis and so on. They also help us prevent and fight cancer, which is a real epidemic of our times. Nowadays, we know from epidemiological studies that there is a connection between health and herbs and spices:

- In India, cancer rates are 2–10 times less frequent than in the United States and Europe.
- In Greece, where rosemary and thyme are widely used, the incidence of cardiac disease is very low.
- In those regions of Spain where saffron is widely used, levels of bad cholesterol (LDL) are lower than in areas where this spice is not eaten.

46. Are there any herbs and spices that are especially good for us?[58, 59]

Almost all herbs and spices have properties that are very positive for our health. However, among those with the best properties, and which have been most studied, we can note the following:

- Thyme, oregano, parsley, celery, basil, mint and rosemary can prevent cancer from spreading by blocking the creation of new blood vessels that feed the tumour (inhibition of angiogenesis).
- Turmeric wards off and fights against any type of cancer. It also protects against Alzheimer's disease and is a powerful anti-inflammatory.
- Ginger: besides being able to inhibit the growth of cancerous cells, a daily infusion alleviates the nausea and vomiting caused by chemotherapy and radiotherapy.

Cinnamon helps control glycaemia, so all diabetics should have some every day.

47. Can I drink tea?[58, 59, 229]

Not only can you drink tea, but you ought to do so every day, whether you are on the Dukan Diet or not, especially if you have cancer – or fear you may one day develop a cancer.

Among the active substances in tea, we should mention epigallocatechin, which is one of the most powerful natural substances to attack the blood vessels in cancerous cells. Unfortunately, when tea leaves are fermented this process destroys the epigallocatechin. So to enjoy the benefits of tea, we have to drink green tea, which not only undergoes no fermentation but also contains greater quantities of this highly protective substance.

Tea is powerful in fighting breast, lung, stomach, bowel and oesophagus cancer. When receiving radiotherapy – for a brain tumour, for example – if drinking tea is combined with the treatment the percentage of tumour cells that respond to the radiotherapy doubles when compared to radiotherapy on its own (i.e. without any tea). Another advantage that tea offers, especially for fans of the Dukan Diet and any other ketogenic diet, is that it increases the food's thermogenic action – drinking tea means more energy has to be used for mastication, digestion and transformation of the nutrients, which allows us to subtly boost our weight loss.

Try and drink your tea without adding any sugar, whether you are dieting or not, because sugar has many harmful effects on our health. If you dislike the taste of strong tea on its own, then you could squeeze in some lemon juice or stir in a cinnamon stick or a teaspoon of ginger or some vanilla. By adding these flavourings to your tea, you are boosting the synergy between the positive action of each type of food as one enhances the beneficial effects of the other on our health. If you don't want to add any flavourings, you can use zero-calorie sweeteners instead.

48. Can I trust the studies available about this type of diet?[230]

Not all published studies are of equal relevance. A clinical case with one patient does not have the same value as a double blind study, in which neither the patients nor the doctors know which group has been given the treatment and which the placebo (the aim is to eliminate any bias when analysing the results). This study will clearly produce results that reflect far more closely what is really happening than the study with a single patient. Indeed, we are able to rank how compelling the evidence is (from top to bottom based on its scientific relevance):

Level I: At least one clinical trial, systematic review or meta-analysis (comparing the results from several studies) correctly carried out.

Level II: More than one comparative trial, cohort studies, case-control or epidemiological studies.

Level III: The opinion of experts or a consensus based on scientific evidence.

Once we are aware of this, we can say that the effects of ketogenic diets have been thoroughly documented in

Level I, II and III studies, which means that they have achieved reliable results, contributing to a scientific consensus that is beyond question.

49. If I can't stand the weekly protein-only day, is there anything I can do?

If you cannot bear not being able to eat a traditional dish with sauce every single day, or if you cannot stand the weekly pure-protein day, here is a very useful tip.

Why not start your protein day just after lunch, a meal that won't consist of proteins only? The protein day then lasts until noon the following day, before your next lunch. This way you do almost 24 hours but it is made more bearable because it is easier to stick to just proteins at breakfast and dinnertime.

However, you won't lose all the weight you ought to lose by following this tip; ideally you should try this twice a week, and not just once as with the standard weekly protein day.

50. On pure protein days, my mouth feels dry and I get bad breath – what can I do?

This happens because of the metabolism of the ketone bodies, which cause dehydration. Furthermore, being very volatile, these bodies get expelled through the nose and through the mouth when we speak. There are two positive aspects about feeling this way: 1) it indicates that you have done your protein day properly; and 2) it encourages you to drink more liquid during the day.

If you want to avoid feeling like this, there are several things you can do:

- Drink zero-calorie drinks at regular intervals.
- Chew on sugar-free chewing-gum as it refreshes the breath, speeds up digestion and lessens the effect of constipation on protein days. Moreover, chewing burns up 1kcal every three minutes, so if we chewed on gum for five hours a day, we would automatically lose an extra 100kcal.
- If you dislike chewing gum, you can buy one of the inexpensive mouth sprays on sale in any supermarket; depending on how often you use the spray, it should last 2–4 weeks. These long-acting products contain xylitol and also act as an antiseptic.

5.

The ketogenic diet and cancer

Or how to die of cancer by following official recommended nutritional guidelines[17, 24, 57, 61–145, 231]

If you look up the website (www.oncosaludable.es) of the Spanish Society of Medical Oncology (SSMO), you will find repeated there the FAO's dietary guidelines, namely: a daily diet consisting of 55–60 per cent carbohydrates, 15–20 per cent proteins and 20–25 per cent lipids, or fats. Yet, as we have already seen, this carbohydrate ratio turns

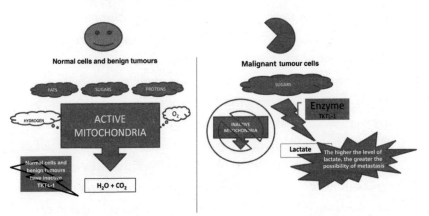

Metabolic differences between normal/benign tumour cells and malignant cancer cells. (Adapted from: *The new anti-cancer diet.* Dr Coy)

out to be actually harmful as it encourages obesity, diabetes, metabolic syndrome, coronary heart disease and cancer. Indeed, cancer metabolism is essentially fuelled by sugar, as the diagram on page 83 demonstrates. For a patient with cancer, there is no better way of feeding their cancer while their healthy cellules die away than to apply these dietary guidelines!

What is further striking is that the FAO and SSMO fail to recommend any foodstuff with a high content of phytochemical, anti-carcinogenic, anti-inflammatory and neuroprotective substances, such as spices, omega-3 rich foods, green tea or dark chocolate. (Phytochemicals are organic chemical compounds found in foods: these substances are not part of the essential nutrients but they can have positive effects on our health.) Yet, a quick glance in the Bibliography (page 231) tells us that already almost 10 years ago Dr Young-Joon Surh, from Seoul National University, published a very important article in the highly prestigious journal *Nature Reviews Cancer*. In it he wrote that *'chemoprevention through eating foods containing phytochemicals is an inexpensive, easily applicable and effective method for controlling and treating cancer'*. Here we should also mention Dr Richard Béliveau from Montreal University who, in 2006, drew together all the research on this topic published over the previous 15 years in specialized journals and wrote up his analysis in language that is clear and accessible to everybody. With so much going on, how can it be possible that doctors and health authorities do not hear about these publications? It is difficult to answer this question without asking yourself who actually stands to gain from such negligence. Why carry on advocating so much sugar and flour while knowing that these foods are too rich for our bodies and, most importantly, that our bodies just don't have the tools or the physiology required to tolerate them? Similarly, phytochemicals are a great help in cooking food to lose weight and to curb the spread of cancer, yet they are not used sufficiently.

Since at present nobody is willing to do it, I am now going to divulge to you what we currently know about this subject and how ketogenic diets can help to prevent and treat cancer.

Glucose and cancer metabolism

A link between sugar and cancer was established by the start of the twentieth century; in Germany, Dr Alfred Braunstein recorded that glycosuria (when sugar is excreted in the urine) stopped in diabetic patients who were developing cancer.

So where had this sugar gone to? IT WAS IN THE CANCEROUS CELL!

Then, using lab-grown cells, it was observed that the cancerous cells used up far more sugar than the healthy ones. Furthermore, and again in Germany, Dr Robert Bierich established that large quantities of lactate were concentrated in the malignant cells, this being a substance that plays a vital role when cancer spreads through body tissue (metastasis) as it pushes the healthy cells to 'commit suicide' (apoptosis), clearing the way for the cancerous cells to take over. Accordingly, as the amount of lactic acid contained in the peritumoural tissue increases, so does the likelihood of metastasis forming. We also know that normal cellular metabolism is aerobic – i.e. the cells need oxygen to turn the glucose into carbon dioxide (CO_2) and water. However, when they cannot get enough oxygen – for example, if we are sprinting – they can switch to anaerobic metabolism, which produces lactate from fermenting the glucose. So if ample oxygen is available, why does cancer produce lactate in laboratory cultures? Because as they become malignant, the cancerous cells are transformed to such an extent that their mitochondria (the powerhouses where energy is really produced in our bodies and responsible for aerobic metabolism) stop working; this means that even if there is oxygen available, the cancerous cells use anaerobic metabolism and therefore have a compelling need to be supplied with glucose. This is the well-known Warburg effect, named after Otto Warburg, the man who discovered it. In the cancerous cells, fermentation of lactates takes place through what is called the expression of *transketolase-like 1* (TKTL1) and the pentose phosphate pathway (conversely, in healthy cells, anaerobic metabolism occurs through what is called the Embden-Meyerhof pathway of anaerobic glycolysis). We can see this phenomenon in the diagram below:

Dogma   **New perspectives**

Change of paradigm

Ketogenic diet

3-hydroxybutyric acid

KIDNEY

Diabetic nephropathy is irreversible

Diabetic nephropathy CAN BE reversible

In 1885, in Germany, Dr Alexander Freund was the first to observe metabolic changes in cancer patients. Of the 70 patients with tumours who were studied, all also had hyperglycaemia and less insulin sensitivity – i.e. the same inflammatory markers as patients suffering from metabolic syndrome! So one could think, intuitively, that by lessening chronic inflammation, insulin sensitivity would be increased while at the same time blood sugar levels would be normalized – which could lower the chances of cancer appearing as well as limiting or putting a check on it developing once it has appeared.

Clinical applications for ketogenic diets with cancer patients

Ketogenic diets help us fight cancer. This hypothesis has been confirmed by a number of laboratory studies on animals and recently by clinical trials and other evidence-based studies. In particular, we should remember the following:

- Clinical trials (Level I evidence) have determined that a ketogenic diet can improve quality of life for very late-stage terminal cancer patients, by reducing inflammatory markers in blood, insulin resistance and hyperglycaemia. The combination of these effects helps to keep in check the undernourishment and cachexia (characterized by loss of weight, muscle atrophy, fatigue and weakness) that the tumour produces. By limiting muscle wasting in this way, the patients regain some energy and are able to enjoy a little physical and social activity, rather than lying prostrate in bed, awaiting their fate.
- New studies appear every day with evidence of how low-carbohydrate diets help and have positive effects on regulating growth in the tumour as well as on regulating the symptoms and deterioration that tumour metabolism produces in patients. Brain tumours, in both children and adults, have been the most closely studied.
- As for these malignant brain tumours, it has been

established that the ketogenic diet does not have any side effects, that it improves patient survival and slows down the tumour's growth rate and the formation of metastases. Basically we can explain how these effects work to contain the tumour because, as we have seen, the mitochondria are inactive in the tumour cells, preventing them from taking energy from the ketone bodies and fatty acids, which instead carry on producing healthy brain cells that can thus maintain their function and normal brain metabolism, whereas the tumour is being deprived of its energy source while this is happening. In a study published this year, Dr Thomas N. Seyfried of Boston College and his working group examined the current state of treatment and how effectively ketogenic diets work on brain tumours. This study even suggests that clinical protocols be put in place to treat malignant brain tumours, consisting of three separate phases: 1) a ketogenic diet to reduce the size and vascularization of the tumour; 2) the possibility of surgery to remove the tumour, after its size and vascularization have been reduced, but also after a 'boundary' has been defined between the tumour and the healthy cells; and 3) continuing with the ketogenic diet during post-operative treatment, so as to act decisively on residual tumour cells post-surgery.

A clinical protocol to treat malignant brain tumours
Phase 1: Ketogenic diet to reduce the size and vascularization of the tumour
Phase 2: Surgery may be carried out on the tumour
Phase 3: The ketogenic diet is continued so as to act on residual tumour cells

By combining the ketogenic diet with eating herbs and spices and taking a little exercise, the benefits from the therapy are boosted considerably, and you stand a better chance of winning the battle against cancer.

To conclude this point, I have drawn up a list below summarizing all that is currently known about the effects of low-carbohydrate ketogenic diets in treating and preventing cancer. I hope that after everything we have just seen, you will understand why, far from protecting us from the effects of cancer, the scientifically dubious guidelines issued by the FAO, SSMO and all official bodies tend instead to play into them as they do not correspond to our physiological and genetic requirements.

Proven effects of a low-carbohydrate diet on the development of cancer and its final results in cancer patients
Malignant tumour cells, using anaerobic metabolism (Warburg effect), encourage resistance to insulin and chronic inflammation
In common with people with metabolic syndrome (obesity, diabetes, high blood pressure) cancer patients tend to be pro-inflammatory and insulin-resistant
Metabolic syndrome increases the risk of the onset of cancer
Low-carbohydrate, ketogenic diets alleviate metabolic syndrome and reduce the risk of cancer appearing

Ketogenic diets are safe and have positive effects for cancer patients, especially for those in advanced stages
Studies conducted in laboratories have established the anti-tumour effects of ketone bodies

Cancer and free radicals: do ketogenic diets encourage oxidation and cancer to develop or do they help fight cancer because of their antioxidant effects?

The current leading theory states that cancers develop primarily because of the damaging, mutagenic effect of free radicals – very reactive and harmful chemical particles derived from oxygen – on our genes (DNA). This means that the more oxidizing the environment, the more the free radicals can proliferate, which increases the chances of a cancer developing. Once the cancer has appeared, it will spread more quickly in an oxidizing environment.

Free radicals develop for the most part in the mitochondria, the body's energy powerhouses, since they are 'working' continuously with oxygen to enable us to breathe. However, these mitochondria do have certain defence mechanisms (i.e. antioxidants) to inhibit the free radicals, in particular vitamins E and C, extracted from what we eat, as well as glutathion (GSH), the main antioxidant that our cells produce. Unfortunately, our eating habits, our lifestyles, smoking and atmospheric pollution all influence our ability to antioxidize, but we shall see that the ketogenic diet actually enables us to retain it.

If, as we have done previously, we study this topic by looking up what is available on Pubmed®, we realize that according to the studies, the ketone bodies produced by ketogenic diets boost GSH synthesis, which in turn boosts the antioxidation function of the mitochondria, inhibiting a greater number of free radicals which in turn protects the DNA from attack. The list below summarizes what else GSH does:

The effects of glutathion (GSH) on the body
GSH is the main antioxidant that our cells secrete
It plays an active part in inhibiting free radicals
It repairs DNA and helps the immune, nervous, respiratory and digestive systems to work properly
It regulates the nitric oxide cycle which plays a fundamental role in maintaining the cardiovascular system (preventing heart attacks)
It helps to prolong the work of the antioxidants we get from our food (vitamins C and E), which destroy the free radicals

6.

The ketogenic diet and diabetes

Or, when in doubt, let's go back to the beginning ... What did our great-grandparents eat?[17, 31–45, 232–235]

Nowadays diabetes, combined with obesity and a poor lifestyle, has taken on truly epidemic proportions. It is now seven times more common than it was in the 1980s. At present there are over 220 million diabetics in the world and this figure is set to rise to over 300 million by 2025 (10 times greater than the 1985 figure!). Clearly something is badly amiss in our society – starting with the nutritional guidelines already mentioned and finishing with the dietary advice issued for treating diabetes.

Conditions associated with diabetes and obesity	
Increased cardiovascular risk	In diabetics, the main cause of mortality is cardiac or cerebral infarction, as diabetics are at a much higher risk of these than the non-diabetic population.

Kidney complaints	Diabetes is the primary cause of kidney failure in Europe and North America.
Eyesight disorders	Diabetic retinopathy is one of the most common causes of blindness and impaired vision in developed countries.
Diabetic foot disorders	Across the world a foot is amputated every 30 seconds. The main reasons for this are blood disorders caused by diabetes.
Erectile dysfunction	Almost half of male diabetics have impotency problems.
Dementia	Diabetics are particularly vulnerable to Alzheimer's disease-type dementia or vascular dementia.

If you are a type 2 diabetic because you are overweight and lead a sedentary lifestyle, or you are pre-diabetic, and you sit there with your arms folded after reading about what lies in store for you, don't even waste your time with this book – just get out there and make the most of what active life you've still got left!

We must not confuse ketosis with acidoketosis

Acidoketosis is the overproduction of ketone bodies, which is bad for our health. Any medical student who doesn't simply want to rely on their professor's notes will have read in their second year Guyton and Hall's *Textbook of Medical Physiology* that '*acidoketosis occurs in pathological conditions such as decompensated diabetes mellitus, prolonged fasting or when there is an abrupt switch from a high-carbohydrate diet to a full-fat diet'*; in other words, when there is no insulin production or when insulin production is malfunctioning. We see that ketogenic diets do nothing of the sort since the proteins we eat and the glucagon hormone released during digestion bring about a slight secretion of insulin, enough to avoid fats accumulating in the body but also enough to prevent acidoketosis. And these mechanisms help us to lose weight by attacking body fat and increasing insulin sensitivity, which is why the diet has a beneficial impact on controlling diabetes.

The effects of a ketogenic diet on type 2 diabetics

Many nutrition, metabolism and diet 'professionals' will try and have you believe that the ketogenic diet is contraindicated for diabetic patients because it will encourage acidoketosis (but we have just seen that this is not true), as well as hypoglycaemia, which is equally untrue.

If we stick with what is currently known scientifically, we see that the proven benefits of this type of diet for diabetic patients include:

- Improved glycaemic balance helping to counterbalance 'ups and downs' in the glycaemia level, whether this be after meals or between meals.
- Improved insulin sensitivity. Type 2 diabetes is characterized by insulin secretion but with impaired

performance. Ketogenic diets improve insulin function, which means that for the same concentration of insulin the results are better for metabolism.

- Reduced glycated haemoglobin levels (HbA1c): at present regularly measuring this level (every six months) is the most reliable parameter for judging the effectiveness of treatment in diabetic patients; the lower the figure (below 6.5 per cent), the more the diabetes is under control. Published studies tell us that this type of diet is the only one where a drop in HbA1c levels has been demonstrated; so this is the type of diet that best helps to regulate diabetes and ward off its devastating side effects.

As we have seen, diabetics are particularly exposed to cardiovascular risk, both from macro-angiopathy (heart attacks, necrosis in the extremities leading to amputation, dementia) as well as from micro-angiopathy (diabetic retinopathy). Given that the diet improves parameters for cardiovascular conditions, does it help reduce the risk of complications and death for diabetics? Yes it does. Among the cardiovascular benefits for diabetic patients that have now been established by publications, the following can be mentioned:

- By comparing a low-fat diet with a (low-carbohydrate) ketogenic diet in obese, diabetic patients it has been possible to prove that the ketogenic diet is more effective not only with regard to weight loss but also in bringing down blood pressure.

- Diabetic patients on a ketogenic diet see an improvement in their lipid (fat) levels, in particular due to a significant increase in good cholesterol (HDL) and a reduction in their triglyceride levels.

In this type of patient, an improvement in controlling blood sugar combined with better control of cardiovascular risk parameters means it is possible, according to the most recent studies, to cut down or even stop long-term medication for 7 out of 10 patients following this type of diet (and a reduction or break in the treatment for cardiovascular risk factors).

Although some critics of this type of diet claim that it results in insulin resistance, as when a person is fasting, studies have proved that the very opposite is the case, as it promotes insulin sensitivity and the synthesis of glycogens (therefore differentiating it from fasting).

Metabolic differences between periods of fasting and the ketogenic diet:

Lipolysis metabolism during a ketogenic diet	Lipolysis metabolism when fasting
• Improved insulin sensitivity	• Insulin resistance
• Glycogens are synthesized spontaneously	• Abolition of glycogen synthesis

To finish off this section, it just remains to say that all these benefits are even more marked in patients who are at risk of becoming diabetic or who are what is termed as pre-diabeties (carbohydrate intolerant): such pre-diabetics can take advantage of all the recorded benefits, avoid taking medication with its possible side effects, and in this way they are 'treating' their 'pre-illness'.

It's tomorrow already: diabetic nephropathy is reversible thanks to the ketogenic diet

I am neither diabetic nor obese nor do I suffer from high blood pressure, or from any other condition. However, a few days after I was born, due to a medical error, I had renal vein thrombosis and one of my kidneys had to be removed. After being monitored for years, I now lead a normal life. However, every lunchtime, as I have my meal in the hospital and down a litre and a half of water, this attracts comments and criticisms from many of my colleagues, who deem such a quantity of water to be bad because it *forces the kidney to hyperfilter*. I do not agree with them. Whether we drink or not, all the blood in our bodies passes through the kidneys every five minutes, give or take a little, and so the cleaner and purer the blood is, the better. What is more, we know from long-term monitoring of people in my situation who are missing a kidney that their remaining kidney does hyperfilter but it does so without causing renal fatigue. During pregnancy, too, the kidneys filter twice as much as they would usually and then three months after the birth they are back working normally again. You will point out that since a woman only has a limited number of pregnancies in her lifetime this amounts to only a short period of time. This is true but it is only true nowadays; during the hunter-gatherer era, women would have had more than 10 pregnancies during their lifetime, so they were in a state of 'hyperfiltration' that was part and parcel of being pregnant for almost 10 years. Yet despite this they didn't suffer from chronic kidney failure – since we, their descendants, are here today to prove it!,

As regards the supposed kidney damage that results from an excess of proteins, a whole series of epidemiological studies prove that there is no such risk in healthy people. Quite the reverse: in an interesting article published a short time ago, Dr M. M. Poplawski and his team from the Mount Sinai School of Medicine in New York have proved, clinically as well as functionally and histologically, that **kidney complaints (including the most serious disorders) resulting from diabetes can be reversible if a ketogenic diet is followed**. Up until now, one of the central dogmas as far as diabetes was concerned was to *regulate glycaemia as strictly as possible to delay the onset of diabetic nephropathy since it is irreversible and its development can only be held in check*. Which meant that before these promising works on the benefits of the ketogenic diet were known about, diabetic patients with kidney disorders scarcely had any choice between a transplant and dialysis. This study calls for further investigation to be carried out, but nonetheless it has raised hopes of a permanent treatment for this sort of disorder, which more often than not eventually results in chronic kidney failure and dialysis. Although the reasons for the reversibility of the nephropathy are not yet completely clear, the authors of this study think that the ketone body called 3–beta-hydroxybutyric acid blocks molecular responses to glucose while having cytoprotective effects, even when there are toxic substances such as free radicals present. If these discoveries were to be confirmed once and for all, ketogenic diets would play a fundamental role in preventing and reversing diabetic foot neuropathy and retinopathy.

To sum up, it is essential for us to understand that the argument about kidneys suffering fatigue when high-protein foods are eaten is not only untrue but the exact opposite is true: ketone bodies help prevent kidney deterioration.

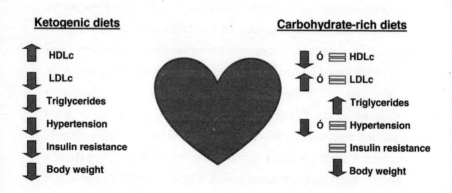

Cardiovascular effects of ketogenic diets compared with carbohydrate-rich diets.

7.

The ketogenic diet, metabolic syndrome and cardiovascular risk

Or there is a dormant fat person within each of us – don't wake them up![15, 17, 192–225]

A number of so-called 'expert' nutritionists advise against ketogenic diets, saying they lead to cardiovascular problems. Their reasons escape me, even more so given that already 10 years ago very positive results for cardiac patients being treated with the Atkins diet had been presented to the American Cardiology Congress. In addition, at the beginning of the 1980s, the United States Department of Agriculture laid down its famous 'food pyramid' model, stating that to prevent and fight obesity a diet should be made up of 50–55 per cent carbohydrates, 15–20 per cent proteins and 20–30 per cent fats. Yet if the 1965 obesity level, when fats comprised 40 per cent of the diet, is compared with the 1991 level, after the current guidelines had been made public, we can see a very significant increase in weight problems and obesity, as well as in triglycerides and atherogenic lipoproteins (VLDL).

Very low density lipoprotein (or 'very bad' cholesterol), VLDLs can lead to atherogenesis, i.e. they may be responsible for atheromas – fatty deposits, plaques – forming in the arteries.

From this we can see that the criticism aimed at ketogenic diets is completely unfounded since these diets turn out instead to be very healthy for people who are obese and/or exposed to cardiovascular risk factors. It is also very instructive (but most worrying!) to discover that diets that are high-carbohydrate (55–60 per cent of total energy) and low-fat, in line with the FAO's guidelines, can actually change the lipid profile by increasing triglycerides and bad cholesterol (LDL), while at the same time bringing down the HDL in patients who had a normal balance before.

The long-term benefits of ketogenic diets, including the Dukan Diet, which has the advantage of reducing fat intake as much as possible (followed for over a year), on patients with cardiovascular risk factors include the following:

- For patients with a high triglyceride level and low levels of good cholesterol (HDL), ketogenic diets bring about a considerable drop in triglycerides and an increase in HDL.
- Compared with high-carbohydrate and low-fat diets, ketogenic diets result in greater loss of body weight and a more marked improvement in cardiovascular risk parameters.

- Although all ketogenic diets improve the lipid profile, low-carbohydrate/high-protein ketogenic diets (like the Dukan Diet) produce a drop in LDL, whereas low-carbohydrate/high-fat diets (like the Atkins diet) lead to a slight increase in LDL. However, this increase is too limited to be harmful, unlike high-carbohydrate diets which instead have an atherogenic effect that encourages cholesterol to build up in the blood vessels, with all the risks of cardiovascular complications that this entails.

- These diets are also beneficial for people with high blood pressure because in the short term (1–3 months) as well as the long term (12 months), they bring about a significant drop in blood pressure, on average greater

In cases of brain trauma...

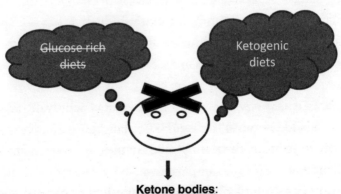

Ketone bodies:
- Improve brain metabolism
- Reduce the production of free radicals
- Protect neurons in the brain

than 10mmHg both for the systolic as well as the diastolic pressure. It would appear that this hypotensive effect is linked to improved insulin sensitivity.

- Moreover, it seems that ketogenic diets may help prevent enlargement of the heart as a result of long-term high blood pressure (hypertensive hypertrophic cardiomyopathy), with the benefits that this brings in terms of reducing the risk of death associated with high blood pressure.

Doctor, I'm not fat! So why do I have high blood pressure?

Strangely enough, almost 4 out of 10 people with a normal weight can have high blood pressure or other disorders connected with metabolic syndrome – insulin resistance, high levels of uric acid, dyslipidemia (a change, often to excess, in the triglyceride level), reproductive physiology disorders, etc. How can this be so? If you ask your doctor, he is likely to say that you are suffering from what is called *essential high blood pressure;* this basically boils down to saying, *essentially*, that he does not know why you have high blood pressure. To disguise our ignorance, we doctors have a habit of attaching odd names to unexplained phenomena! So, for example, nowadays we use three terms to describe high blood pressure (other than *essential*):

- Idiopathic: from the Greek *pathos* meaning 'suffering, trial, illness', and *idios,* 'pertaining to yourself'. It is as if you were being told: 'You are doing what we call *high blood pressure yourself*'!

- Primary: a term used to denote that we do not know the real reasons for a disorder (it is *'secondary'* when the reasons are known); we say of the disorder that it *exists in itself* (primary or unknown reason).
- Cryptogenic: another term from the Greek, meaning 'of hidden (*crypto*) origin (*genesis*)'.

If you were to ask 100 doctors about the most common cause of high blood pressure, 95 of them will give an irrelevant answer, citing *essential high blood pressure*. Since they don't know what causes it, they can only give you some medication to lower it. On the other hand, among the five doctors who have the correct answer we can name Dr Gerald Reaven, a cardiologist at the Stanford University School of Medicine in California. This well-known endocrinologist was the first to identify metabolic syndrome. The remaining four doctors, who, like me, know the most common cause of high blood pressure, are those doctors who have read Dr Reaven's works and have put them into practice with their patients!

Almost 20 years ago, Dr Reaven discovered that by cutting down their carbohydrate intake, his patients with high blood pressure – slim *and* obese – would see their readings become normal or register a considerable drop. And this would happen without any medication. This can be explained physiologically because a high-carbohydrate diet produces high insulin concentration in the blood, which has three effects that drive up blood pressure and keep it high:

1. Insulin boosts re-absorption of sodium (salt) in the kidneys and this enters the bloodstream, pushing up blood pressure.
2. A body that expels less salt (sodium) needs to re-absorb more water in the kidneys (liquid retention) in order to dilute this excess sodium, thereby increasing blood pressure.
3. Lastly, a major effect that insulin has is that it activates the sympathetic nervous system to keep us in a state of vigilance (flight, fight, stress, etc.), resulting in a sustained increase in blood pressure.

Now that we know the reasons for essential high blood pressure, if you have high readings why don't you try, under medical supervision, a low-carbohydrate diet for 2–3 weeks (phases 1 and 2 of the Dukan Diet are ideal for this) and monitor your readings. You will see your blood pressure return to normal and if you opt for this lifestyle, you may even be able to cut down or give up your medication.

Curiously, in hunter-gatherer tribes, the Eskimos and all peoples who eat few carbohydrates, it is the elderly who have the lowest blood pressure readings. In these groups, there is no such thing as high blood pressure, unlike in our societies where it is the elderly and the middle-aged who take the most pills to treat what is now such a common complaint.

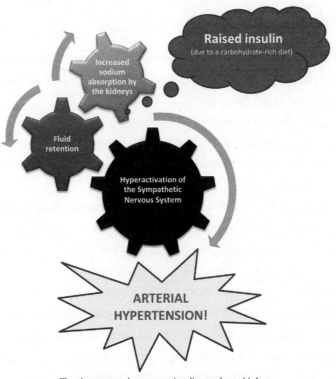

The three ways that excess insulin produces high
blood pressure (arterial hypertension)

The Spanish Mediterranean ketogenic diet and cardiovascular health

As Spain is one of the countries where the Mediterranean
diet – a diet for which all the health benefits are known
– holds sway Dr Pérez-Guisado and his team at the
University of Córdoba, leading researchers in ketogenic
diets, have developed a ketogenic diet that includes the
four typical components of Spanish gastronomy: fish,

olive oil, red wine and salad. This diet is split up into the following:

- unlimited protein intake, with particular emphasis on fish; meat, eggs, seafood, cheese and poultry are also allowed
- red wine, maximum 200–400ml a day
- carbohydrates, 30 grams eaten as salad and vegetables
- extra virgin olive oil, 30ml minimum a day
- herbs and spices used to season salads
- at least 3 litres of water a day, and no more than two cups of coffee or tea per day
- calorie-free sweeteners are also permitted

After a three-month study, this ketogenic diet proved to be as effective as other ketogenic diets with regard to weight loss and improved cardiovascular risk parameters, expressed in particular through a drop in systolic and diastolic blood pressure, lower triglyceride and bad cholesterol (LDL) levels, and an increase in good cholesterol (HDL).

So we have here an interesting option that obese patients with cardiovascular risk factors could think of trying if they are loath to give up the principles of the Mediterranean diet and its pleasures, such as a daily glass of wine and salad.

8.

The ketogenic diet, high levels of uric acid and gout

Or how to prevent and best treat gout by cutting down on carbohydrates[236–239]

You've got gout? Or maybe you know some one who does?

If this is the case, then I imagine that your doctor, apart from his pills and potions, will have advised you to cut out the following as far as possible: seafood, offal, meat, duck, goose, pork, bacon, fish, mushrooms, asparagus, tomatoes, etc. Am I right? The good news is that scientific studies have shown that such a restricted diet, far from preventing and effectively treating this disorder, tends instead to encourage the onset of further attacks. The bad news is that your doctor probably does *not yet* know about this so he is still depriving you of the foods you enjoy so much – while at the same time possibly encouraging new bouts of gout to develop!

Purines are found in foods with high nitrogen levels, such as meat and cooked meat products, offal, fish and seafood. We are going to see how a low-purine diet (precursors to uric acid) can help worsen this disease and lead to more attacks than a high-purine diet.

Our friend Dr Reaven provided us with an explanation for all this years ago: too much insulin in the blood results in large quantities of uric acid being re-absorbed in the

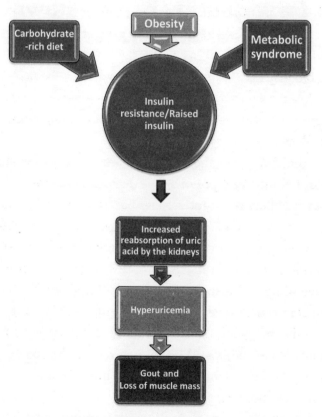

How uric acid builds up in the blood and leads to gout

kidneys instead of being eliminated in the urine. However, the result is that a diet that cuts out high-purine foods will be high in carbohydrates. These carbs will help increase our insulin resistance and boost the process whereby uric acid gets re-absorbed in the kidneys (given that 95 per cent of the uric acid produced by the body is due to production in the liver and the diet has no impact on the liver).

It is quite apparent that when there are high levels of uric acid in the blood, the decisive factor is that the uric acid gets re-absorbed by the kidneys and goes back into the bloodstream instead of being expelled in the urine, as has been proved by several research teams since Gerald Reaven and his team produced the first publications on this subject in the 1990s.

One of the advantages of a low-carbohydrate diet is that gout medication can be avoided – along with its many side effects. As we have seen throughout this book, a low-carbohydrate diet will also help improve our general state of health while at the same time lowering our risk of developing the most common chronic diseases.

9.

The ketogenic diet, Alzheimer's disease, epilepsy, traumatic brain injuries

Or how too much sugar causes inflammation in our neurones that will make us forget everything[17, 240–248]

Since 1921, when Dr Russell Wilder of the Rochester Mayo Clinic, USA, successfully treated epileptic children who did not respond to medication with a high-fat, low-carbohydrate ketogenic diet (eggs, bacon, meat, fish, oil, hamburgers, cheese etc.), there have been many variations on this type of diet which have all turned out to be most effective in treating the condition without any serious side effects, and in significantly lowering the number of epileptic attacks.

At present, the main cause of dementia is Alzheimer's disease, characterized by cerebral atrophy of the frontal, temporal and parietal lobes, neurofibrillary tangles and senile plaques. As far as metabolism goes, there is a reduction in the brain's metabolism since it has less capacity to use glucose as a source of energy. However, published studies have confirmed that to maintain brain activity in this type of patient, ketone bodies could provide an alternative to glucose. In some studies, the patients were divided into two groups: one was given a placebo and the other tablets with medium chain fatty acids or medium chain triglycerides. Compared with the placebo group, it was noticed that the patients who had received the ketogenic treatment showed a marked improvement when tested for memory and attention. So this treatment is an option to be considered both for guarding against Alzheimer's disease and other types of dementia resulting from changes in brain glucose metabolism and its early-stage treatment.

Studies, backed up by cerebral imagery, have confirmed that there is a connection between obesity and an increased risk of dementia and Parkinson's disease. Yet, following a low-calorie diet is all it takes to reduce neurological risk factors. Experimental studies carried out on animals inoculated with Parkinson's disease have shown that if calorie intake is cut, motor skills improve and at the same time neuronal loss in the brain's black substance (*substantia nigra*) is reduced, which slows down the development of the disease.

As a rule, the theory of hormesis is used to explain the benefits of low-calorie diets on the brain. When a minor stress response is triggered, this in turn activates metabolic and genetic pathways that improve the brain's performance. To understand this mechanism better, we should see hormesis as having similar positive effects on the brain as physical exercise has on the muscles and heart; physical effort puts our muscle system under stress, which activates appropriate mechanisms so that the body adapts to this stress and performs better. Restricting calorie intake also has an antioxidizing effect which gives this diet additional positive impact.

Low-calorie diets and ketogenic diets share two features: 1) limited carbohydrate intake that in itself produces neuroprotective action, as has been widely proved; and 2) an offsetting increase in ketone bodies.

Insofar as ketogenic diets are usually combined with physiological calorie restriction, the benefits of low-calorie diets get added to the intrinsic positive effects of ketogenic diets.

Sometimes children and young adults suffer cranio-encephalic trauma. Although such trauma can sometimes be fatal, in cases where the victims survive permanent neurological damage can be avoided through the timely administration of suitable treatment. We know that administering glucose early on to patients with cranio-encephalic trauma is harmful, since it inhibits physiological ketogenesis and its protective effects on the brain while at the same time insulin levels and lactic acid production go up. Consequently, any glucose intake must be stopped for patients at risk of suffering irreversible damage. What is more, the ketone bodies' cerebral metabolism improves metabolic performance in the mitochondria and boosts the release of energy as ATP (adenosine triphosphate is the molecule that, in the biochemistry of known living organisms, transports the energy required for the chemical reactions in metabolism), while reducing the production of free radicals. This all goes to confirm, if confirmation were needed, that ketone bodies have a neuroprotective effect.

As regards the side effects of ketogenic diets, we should mention: 1) dehydration, especially in children who do not drink enough; 2) vomiting and nausea; 3) constipation, and 4) hypoglycaemia, though this is slight and quickly corrected. The positive effects therefore seem to outweigh the undesirable ones. This type of diet is recommended for all patients with central nervous system disorders such as epilepsy and other less common but equally disabling syndromes. And should these side effects seem nasty to you, then what can we say about the drugs prescribed to treat this type of condition, whose effects at the lowest end of the scale range from vomiting to headaches but can include loss of libido and sexual desire? So it seems best to try the diet first!

10.

Addicted to carbohydrates?

The toxic truth about sugar![249–251]

Our consumption of carbohydrates and sugar has tripled in the past 50 years, leading to nothing less than a pandemic of obesity and other complaints. This situation is alarming as it has been calculated that eating too much sugar may be responsible for 35 million deaths a year, through cancer, heart attacks or diabetes.

It is often thought that obesity is the source of all diseases. This is not entirely accurate as 2 out of 10 obese people have no metabolic disorder at all and are able to lead a normal life. On the other hand, 4 out of 10 people with a normal weight develop metabolic syndrome (diabetes, high blood pressure, cholesterol and triglyceride disorders, high levels of uric acid, cardiac diseases and fatty liver). Excessive sugar consumption can explain all this. So it is just as vital to avoid becoming obese as it is to follow a low-carbohydrate diet, even if you are slim! For our cells, chronic exposure to sugar is in fact so harmful that it can be compared to excessive and chronic exposure to alcohol, as is shown in the table below.

Chronic exposure to alcohol	Chronic exposure to sugar
Haematological disorders	–
Hydroelectrolytic disorders	–
High blood pressure	High blood pressure
Cardiac dilation	–
Cardiomyopathy	Myocardial infarction
Dyslipidemia	Dyslipidemia
Pancreatitis	Pancreatitis
Obesity	Obesity
Malnutrition	Malnutrition linked to obesity
Hepatic disorders (Alcoholic steatohepatitis)	Hepatic disorders (Non-alcoholic steatohepatitis)
Alcoholic cirrhosis	Non-alcoholic cirrhosis
Liver cancer	Liver cancer
Foetal alcohol syndrome	–
–	Tooth decay
Gout	Gout
Addiction	Addiction

You would never have imagined that sugar could be so harmful, would you? There is a simple explanation why it is: the only sugars our ancestors came across were those found in fruit – only available for a few months a year and in limited quantities – and in honey that was jealously 'guarded' by the bees. Our genes and our cells are not designed to continually consume and be exposed to sugar.

The more carbohydrates we eat, the more our bodies demand

Our permanent and compulsive desire to eat high-carbohydrate foods packed with refined sugars is now so widespread that a word has been coined in the USA and the UK to describe this new addiction: *chocoholic*. But what is it that makes us so addicted to carbohydrates?

Consuming high-carbohydrate foods forces the pancreas to produce a large quantity of insulin. In turn, the insulin encourages this large quantity of sugar – which suddenly enters the bloodstream from the intestines, inducing hyperglycaemia – to quickly get right to the heart of our cells, which results in a temporary drop in our blood sugar level (hypoglycaemia). This phenomenon reaches a peak a few hours after a meal, triggering a 'hunger and desire to eat high-carb foods' response in the brain so that the optimum blood sugar level can be re-established, which ends up creating the vicious circle that means that:

The more carbohydrates we eat at each meal, the greater our desire to eat more carbs a few hours after we've eaten!

Now do you understand why, after a siesta following a hearty meal comprising bread, starchy foods, rice, pasta, potatoes or other such foods, you long for something a 'bit sweet'? This happens also because, in general, you are 'addicted' to carbohydrates and need to eat some every day.

On the other hand, if you put the Dukan Diet principles into practice, or those of other ketogenic diets, your body will not secrete large quantities of insulin after each meal; your blood sugar level will not yo-yo and not only will your brain not 'force' you to take in sugar barely a few hours after you have finished eating but, quite the opposite, your brain will register satiety for a longer period.

A fortnight without junk food or sugar

High-fat and high-carb foods work on the brain like a drug, similar to cocaine or heroin. Studies show that eating high-fat, high-carb foods packed with calories produces a massive release of dopamine in our brains akin to the effect of taking drugs. Then, to achieve the same levels of dopamine and pleasure, we have to keep eating ever greater quantities of this type of food, which is why we get so addicted to high-sugar diets – to get the same pleasure, the 'dose' has to be increased from day to day!

Another astonishing discovery is that such foods are said to have addictive effects that last six times longer than those of soft drugs; it takes two weeks of abstinence from sugar for our dopamine level to return to normal. This will help you better understand why the Dukan Diet can prove a little difficult to follow for the first six or seven days. However, once you have 'come off' eating junk food and sugars every day, not only will the diet seem far easier but you will also feel euphoric, full of energy and you'll sleep better – just a few examples of the diet's many advantages that we won't revisit here.

11.

Can you use a book to lose weight?

How much can you trust a book? Is there really no risk? Does it work?[252–259]

S ince Dr Dukan brought out his book *The Dukan Diet*, thereby helping millions of people to shed their unwanted pounds – simply, inexpensively and effectively – while at the same time giving them the means to remain at a healthy weight for the rest of their lives, many doctors and nutritionists have attempted to discredit the diet, stating in essence 'that you can't lose weight with a book; not only is it useless, but it is dangerous'. And yet, if we take a look at the studies published on this subject, we see that the method used by Dr Dukan is not only simple, easy to follow and risk-free, but, most importantly, it is the most effective method for anyone who wants to lose their surplus pounds and not put them back on again over the long term. Indeed, as various independent teams of researchers from the United States, Canada and northern Europe have confirmed, successfully tackling obesity depends on the following key factors:

1. Self-motivation

The central factor is *becoming aware* that we want to lose weight; we have to make it possible for ourselves to follow a slimming programme. It is not about being determined to lose weight for the doctor or nutritionist whom we consult once a week or fortnight because we have to give an account of our efforts, but rather because we have fully taken on board the idea that losing weight is good for our health.

2. Knowing about foods

Knowing which foods we can and can't eat; being thoroughly acquainted with them helps us to reinforce proactive behaviour around our weight loss.

3. Understanding that the effectiveness of a diet does not depend on calorie counting

There is very little leeway here. We need to take in so many calories per day – for example, 2,000 calories for an adult male. It is impossible to reduce this intake without feeling very tired or famished. Moreover, counting the calories for each food is very complicated. Indeed, it has been proved that diets based on calorie counting do not work. Two years after starting this type of diet 95 per cent of patients have regained all the weight they lost. What is more, with this sort of diet most of the weight lost is down to muscle mass loss. Conversely, Dukan-type diets, where you can eat as much as you want of the *foods that are allowed*, mean that you lose weight from your fat and not your muscles, as well as keeping up your spirits while avoiding the anxiety that comes from having your daily calorie intake restricted.

4. Controlling the diet yourself

It has been proved that being able to set your own weekly diet programme yourself – two days of pure proteins followed by two days of proteins and vegetables, for example – is one of the most reliable indicators for a diet being successful, and for maintaining a healthy weight over the long term.

5. Planning for changes in eating habits

Phase 3 of the Dukan Diet ensures that the patient gradually internalizes healthy eating habits that will enable them to have a better relationship with food, over the long term and for life. This is all planned well in advance and is discussed at the start of the diet.

6. Flexibility and correcting eating lapses

For a diet to be effective over time, it has to be flexible so that it can be adapted to each individual's lifestyle and needs. It also needs to provide you with the right tools to compensate for any eating lapses that happen, say, when you are out with others. From phase 3, the Dukan Diet allows you to enjoy what it calls 'celebration meals'. In return, it sets three non-negotiable lifetime rules from phase 4 onwards: a daily walk plus no lifts or escalators, daily oat bran, and one pure protein day a week.

To date the studies available show that any diet that satisfies these six aspects (and the Dukan Diet is one of them) works better than diets based on periodic supervision by experts in nutrition. In fact, as far as mental attitude and motivation are concerned, forcing yourself to 'lose weight' for the sake of 'being accountable to somebody else' will end up sapping willpower and will result in the very opposite effect of the one intended: *anxiety, increased high-carbohydrate food intake and the regain of any weight lost.*

The table below shows that the Dukan Diet meets all the criteria for an effective, risk-free diet that you can follow on your own.

Checklist to assess if a diet is feasible without any outside support
1. A diet based, from the start, on clearly defined phases that you the patient can understand
2. A diet that sets out which foods you can and cannot eat
3. A diet based on metabolism being controlled by insulin antagonistic hormones (this type of metabolism guards against and avoids side effects such as hypoglycaemia, protein undernutrition, etc.)
4. A varied, flexible diet that includes a programme which can be adapted to fit each individual and takes eating lapses and variations into account
5. A diet that is not a low-calorie diet

You will have realized that if you yourself are not proactive about taking care of your health then nobody else is going to do it for you! This is where the Dukan method really comes into its own as it puts the emphasis on you managing your dieting yourself, working from a very clear awareness of what you are about. Morever, we should make clear that the Dukan method may be followed in part with help from a coach, who can support the dieter whenever they feel discouraged or find the going tough. Lastly, there is an online forum where everyone can share their successes, find answers to their questions and help other people.

With their work, Dr Frisch and his team from Bonn University in Germany have proved that, when a person follows a weight-loss diet, being able to **count on support or monitoring, from a coach or from internet forums, helps the person not only to lose weight but also to keep enjoying the advantages that result from it and not regain over time the pounds they've shed**. By comparing a high-carbohydrate diet (like those advocated by the WHO and the FAO) and a low-carbohydrate diet (Dukan type), his team also proved that, of the two, the low-carbohydrate diet achieves the best results. This is true for weight loss over the short and long term (greater loss of fat and a more marked reduction in wrist measurements), and it also improves cardiovascular risk parameters (lower triglyceride levels and systolic blood pressure without any drop in good cholesterol (HDL)).

12.

Can we compare diets based on protein sachets or bars with the Dukan Diet?

Are there any advantages in using sachets?[1-4, 16, 260]

In the 1970s, a diet based on liquid protein sachets appeared in the United States and resulted in the death of more than 60 people. These sachets were withdrawn from sale but without any proper inquiry being held into what caused these fatalities. However, over 30 years later, the idea of a protein sachet-based ketogenic diet has made a powerful comeback. This diet has nothing in common with a diet based on natural foods, like Dukan or Atkins.

The arguments put forward by those who defend these protein sachet-based diets include the following:

1. *'The protein sachets used nowadays are safe phar-maceutical products that pose no risk to health and bear no relation to the sachets that were on sale in the 1970s.'*

This statement is not completely accurate: on the one hand, it is impossible to confirm that a pharmaceutical product is totally safe; all medication has side effects, some are harmless, others are serious (the third leading cause of death in the United States is the adverse effects of prescription drugs). On the other hand, since there has never been an investigation into the precise reasons why people died in the 1970s after using these protein sachets, it is impossible to confirm that there are no comparable risks with the current sachets (the absence of proof is not the proof of absence).

2. A staunch proponent of the protein sachet-based diet, about which he has written a book, *The Protein Diet*, is the Catalan nutritionist Dr Molins who states that '*the advantage of using protein sachets over normal foods is that the sachets contain high biological-value proteins and very little fat*'. Consequently he believes that '*these sachets are healthier and better for the body than a Dukan type of diet, where natural foods from plants and animals are always eaten*'.

However, Dr Molins' argument has several flaws (as I have had the pleasure of discussing with him at length on a nutrition blog where I have pointed out his mistakes to him):

• High biological-value, high-protein foods, i.e. foods that contain the amino acids we need to form our proteins, are none other than foods of animal origin – meat and fish. So we have absolutely no need for any artificial products to improve our dietary intake. In other words, in order to work properly over the course of evolution, our bodies have developed their amino acid requirements to fit around the plants and animals naturally available. This means that, scientifically speaking, using protein sachets as food supplements or as a substitute for real food offers no advantage whatsoever.

- If these protein sachets are so good and better than natural foods, then why aren't they prescribed to patients for life? This type of diet is split into various phases, starting with the initial phase when only the sachets and a few vegetables are eaten, ending with the final phase (after around 1–2,000 euros have been spent in the meantime on consultations and sachets), when we are told that *we don't need the sachets any more because we now know how to eat healthily.* This just emphasizes how absurd and inconsistent this system is, as it amounts to saying: 'You'll start your diet off by eating the best and most healthy thing there is (protein sachets), but after some time you'll go back to a diet based on foods of lower quality (natural foods).'

- Dr Molins acknowledges himself in his book that: '*patients over 65, people with diabetes, heart disease or high blood pressure on thiazide-type medication, patients on corticosteroids, or suffering from cancer or autoimmune diseases must not follow my diet* [etc.].' If these sachets are so good for our health, why are there so many contraindications?

As I have clarified throughout this book, any ketogenic diet based on natural foods, such as the Dukan Diet, may not only be used by patients with many different conditions – diabetes, high blood pressure, cancer, etc. – but, what is more, these patients stand to gain hugely in terms of their health and physiology. The same cannot be said of the protein sachets diet, contraindicated for just about any patient with a chronic disorder.

Lastly, and especially important in these times of austerity, it is interesting to note that for the price of 4–5 protein sachets, which is the dose required for a single day, you can buy the book on the Dukan method and follow this diet happily at home, at little expense and without running any risk. Instead of buying protein sachets, you could spend your money on healthier, more appealing things, like eating natural foods! Moreover, if buying these sachets is supposedly justified because they come with personalized, medical supervision (needless to say, by paying for consultations), then your GP can offer you this supervision – although the Dukan Diet does not strictly speaking require any – and supervision that is free of charge, reliable and disinterested, since the GP's job is specifically to promote healthy living and tackle obesity and the chronic diseases associated with it.

13.

The Dukan Diet and ketogenic diets: 10 myths tested against reality

Myth no. 1: The Dukan Diet is full of fats and proteins.
Reality no. 1: The Dukan Diet is a ketogenic diet, essentially low-carbohydrate and high-protein, during its first phase and a little less in the second. In each of its phases, it is low-fat.

Myth no. 2: The Dukan Diet is anything but a natural diet!
Reality no. 2: Because of what it comprises, the Dukan Diet is very close to our ancestors' diet and so, by extension, to the food that our genes are accustomed to; it is precisely this way of eating that helped the human race survive difficult periods of time, when food was scarce.

Myth no. 3: The Dukan Diet causes kidney stones.
Reality no. 3: The Dukan Diet does not cause kidney stones any more than a normal diet. To eliminate any risk of renal lithiasis (stones), all you actually need to do is drink 2–3 litres of water a day.

Myth no. 4: The Dukan Diet is not good if you are diabetic.

Reality no. 4: The Dukan Diet is excellent for diabetics since it lowers insulin resistance and improves glycaemic control, while at the same time reducing cardiovascular risk markers and complications arising from the diabetes.

Myth no. 5: The Dukan Diet attacks muscle mass.

Reality no. 5: The Dukan Diet will burn away your fat but it will not touch any muscle mass.

Myth no. 6: The Dukan Diet is carcinogenic.

Reality no. 6: The Dukan Diet, like all ketogenic diets, deprives the cancer of its only fuel, glucose; this has been proved in the numerous studies into the benefits of ketogenic diets in treating cancer. Ketosis arrests the development of tumours and limits the risk of metastases.

Myth no. 7: The Dukan Diet is unsuitable for children and teenagers.

Reality no. 7: The Dukan Diet is suitable for children with epilepsy who do not respond to medication, which proves that children and teenagers can follow it. Furthermore, publications show that ketogenic diets produce very good results with children who have brain tumours.

Myth no. 8: The Dukan Diet leads to liver disorders.

Reality no. 8: Far from being bad for your liver, by banning fats and alcohol the Dukan Diet brings relief to the liver and helps cut down the amount of fat accumulated in the organ (steatosis).

Myth no. 9: The Dukan Diet is not recommended if you have cardiac complaints.

Reality no. 9: The Dukan Diet improves lipid profile and blood pressure levels; if you have cardiac complaints it could not be more suitable.

Myth no. 10: You do not eat anything healthy on the Dukan Diet.

Reality no. 10: For a few days, the Dukan Diet starts off with proteins, the only vital food, then it adds vegetables, which are essential, then fruit, which is important, next bread, which is useful, then cheese, which is nutritional, starchy foods, which are energy giving and finally celebration meals for pure pleasure. In four phases, it takes in the complete range of healthy foods.

Appendix

A few letters in reply to 'my dear expert' nutritionists, fierce critics of the Dukan Diet

Letter to the Review and Positioning Group of the Spanish Association of Dieticians and Nutritionists (GREP-AEDN) about the Dukan 'diet' or 'method' (March 2011).

Dear GREP-AEDN members,

I am writing to share some observations with you about the manifesto you published in March 2011 attacking the Dukan Diet. To quote your own words, you *'strongly advise against the "method" or "diet" that M. Dukan puts forward . . . because it is ineffective, misleading and potentially dangerous. This opinion is based on the . . . following considerations concerning this "diet" or "method" '*:

1. No scientific basis
'No Spanish or international scientific database . . . contains any study that refers to this diet and which would prove that it is effective and safe.'

'The author's word and the personal experiences of those who have used it . . . are of no value from the point of view of scientific proof and public health.'

My observations about this argument: You yourselves say that *'no . . . scientific database contains any study that refers to this diet'*. So how do you know that it is bad? If there is no study about it, we cannot know whether it is a good or a bad diet. In other words, the absence of proof is not the proof of absence, and by letting it be known that since nothing has been published in favour of this diet (but nothing against it either, as you acknowledge) then it has to be bad, your reasoning is fallacious. What is more. if *'the author's word'* is not *'scientific proof'*, should we then believe that yours on the other hand is? Indeed, when advising against this diet, your word is the only proof you provide.

On the other hand, if I say to you that as a surgeon I am going to operate on you and perform 'a Campillo', you can search the databases all you like but you will find no reference anywhere pertaining to the operation in question. However, if I were to tell you that I am going to carry out a left colectomy followed by closure of the rectal stump and terminal colostomy, i.e. a Hartmann operation, you will find out about the type of surgery you are about to undergo far more easily. What I mean is that the Dukan Diet is a *ketogenic diet, a high-protein, low-carbohydrate and low-fat diet.* The name has not been associated with the diet for long enough for articles mentioning the name Dukan to have been published. This is not the case for the Atkins diet, about which there are many publications, since it became popular in the 1980s. If you had therefore shown more of this scientific rigour of which you speak, you would have searched the databases for terms such as: 'ketogenic diets', 'low-carbohydrate diets', 'effects of ketogenic diets', 'complications from low-carbohydrate diets', etc. Then, indeed, you could take a properly informed stance and explain to the general public what is currently known about this topic.

My conclusion about the GREP-AEDN's first argument: The criticism mentioned here completely lacks scientific rigour; it is not built on any solid argument and is full of contradictions. You make do with the name of the thing (the Dukan Diet), while knowing nothing at all about the said diet. Your flawed thinking is based only on your own word and not on scientific reality.

2. 'This diet has features that as far as diets are concerned amount to a sham.'
To me this is the most ridiculous argument of all; just because something has a set of characteristics that are typical of a certain class of objects does not mean that it irrefutably belongs to this group. By induction, you have made an error here and I am really sorry to have to say this to you. It is possible that some pseudo-diets fulfil these criteria, but this does not mean that all diets that meet these criteria are a sham, especially when we are well aware of the role that, for example, slogans and

marketing play nowadays to try and attract customers. In actual fact, your indictment aims to do nothing other than to win back the customers you have lost to the Dukan method. This is the law of the capitalist economy and the role of advertising. And taking on a book that only costs a few euros is that much more difficult.

If you wanted to prove that this diet is a sham, you should have used scientific arguments to demonstrate that it is based on deceit. Using them, you could have alerted the general public to how the diet fulfils these criteria and invited everyone to assess the suitability of their diet. I have studied all the scientific literature published on ketogenic diets and I can tell you quite definitely that at the present time there is nothing sham about them and that they are not bad for our health, quite the opposite in fact.

As for the eight criteria you use to define fraudulent diets, which according to you the Dukan Diet fulfils, I disagree with you about the following points:

- You state that this diet promises *'quick'* (characteristic no. 1) and *'miraculous'* (characteristic no. 2) results, which is not true. Indeed, although there is some rapid weight loss at the start, the whole programme comprises four phases, and the third one lasts *'five days for every pound lost'*, i.e. 100 days if you have shed 20 pounds (almost a whole year if you have lost 50–60 pounds), and this does not take into account the time spent beforehand losing those pounds. So here is a diet that seems neither quite so *'quick'* nor *'miraculous'* as all that, and Dr Dukan himself acknowledges in his books that to keep on top of things *'you will have to do a day of pure proteins every week for the rest of your life to avoid putting weight back on'*. True, he does also admit that this weekly pure protein day will allow you to enjoy two 'celebration meals' a week without regaining weight, but his promises stop there. If you want to further indulge yourself, then you'll need to do more protein days in the week or else you'll put the weight back on. Dr Dukan says all this.

- Nor does Dr Dukan advocate any *'health products with extraordinary properties'* (characteristic no. 6). He does recommend eating oat bran every day as a source of filling fibre. There is nothing here about fibre in all its forms that we do not already know.

- This diet *'exaggerates the scientific truth about a food'* (characteristic no. 5). I do not see what you are referring to here, since the diet does not ascribe any magical properties whatsoever to anything at all. Indeed, the diet is based around alternating between ketogenic phases and normal phases. The physiology for ketogenesis has been fully established in many publications. Perhaps you have been led to see exaggeration here because you are ill- acquainted with the subject area. I would therefore recommend that you read the scientific articles published in journals or read this book.

- Characteristic no. 8 states that this diet *'contains claims that run counter to those of reputable health bodies'*. Here is a pronouncement typifying the 'principle of authority', or as I call it 'health professionals dressed up as sheriffs'. I had assumed that this principle, which held sway until the Renaissance, had long been abolished. Not to mention that science could never make any headway if it did not challenge established knowledge and learning. Let's take as an example the difficulties that the 16th-century barber-surgeon Ambroise Paré came up against. Had he not stood up to the establishment, he would never have been able to lay down the principles that still govern how wounds and amputations are treated and dealt with today.

So we see that this diet corresponds to virtually none of the characteristics that you wrongly and rather hastily attribute to it.

My conclusion about the GREP-AEDN's second argument: I hope, for the good of the Spanish public, that this manifesto has nothing to do with the people in charge of the AEDN. Because if this were the case they would be guilty here of a serious lack of professionalism and scientific rigour, as we have just seen. The Dukan Diet does not fulfil any of the criteria that characterize sham diets; moreover, your reasoning makes it impossible to establish whether there is any truth or not in an argument. You are confusing the mirage of induction and reality here.

3. Wrongly attributing the ability to cause weight loss to dietary proteins.

With this argument, dear GREP-AEDN members, once again your line of reasoning is mistaken in the way I have already outlined in the first point of this letter and which was summed up in the 1980s by Douglas Altman, professor of biostatistics and editing director of *The British Medical Journal*, when he said that: '*the absence of proof is not the proof of absence*'. As you yourselves stated in a review dating from 2003, '*there is no proof to show that increased protein content helps with weight loss*'. However, the article to which you were then referring said literally: '*there is not sufficient proof to make recommendations for or against low-carbohydrate diets*', which is something very different to what you state in your text. In addition, since 2003 water has passed under the bridge and many other reviews, far more complete as they are based on a much greater number of articles, have since been published. Today there is a sufficient body of evidence to recommend these diets without fear at all. On this subject, I suggest you read the review published in 2011 by Dr Joaquín Pérez-Guisado of the University of Córdoba: 'Ketogenic diets: additional benefits to weight loss and unfounded side effects.'

As for the other article you refer to, published in 2009 in the *New England Journal of Medicine* by Dr Sacks et al., if you have read it you must have seen that it does not deal with ketogenic diets at all since, of the four diets examined, the one that is lowest in carbohydrates still contains 35 per cent, and therefore is not in the least comparable with the Dukan Diet. I do not know whether this escaped you, whether you did not read this article or whether the sole objective in mind was to vilify, by lying if necessary.

As for the argument according to which 'high intake of dietary proteins . . . is not exempt from risk. On the one hand, monitoring what 22,944 adults ate over 10 years has shown that eating prolonged low-carbohydrate and high-protein diets is associated with an increase in the overall mortality rate. A study carried out on 85,168 women over 26 years and 44,548 men over 20 years . . . has reached the same conclusions.' Including these articles does not seem very honest to me because if you read them right through you will see that the figures for mortality are given as *hazard ratios* – i.e. in terms of relative risk, which makes interpreting them very tricky and leads us to believe that there are some very substantial discrepancies between one diet and the other. However, in reality, if we convert them as *absolute risk* (as honesty would demand if we want the general public to understand things as they really are), we then see in both studies that, of the 1,000 patients following a diet different from the one you criticize, 10 died over this period, as against 11 or 12 in the group on the low-carbohydrate diet, i.e. the difference is so slight that in reality it becomes imperceptible. Moreover, Fung's study states that 'low-carbohydrate diets based on plant products show a lower mortality rate'. However, you do not quote this either in your argument.

Finally, I will refer you once again to Professor

Pérez-Guisado's 2011 review and suggest you read it so that you stop spreading the idea of side effects that do not exist.

My conclusion about the GREP-AEDN's third argument: To formulate this argument, you have relied on lies and on concealing information, and have not looked at the most recent scientific literature on the subject. Revealed here, these lies rob you of any scientific credibility. Whenever in the future you talk about mortality rates, I would urge you to have the honesty to do so in terms of absolute risk or natural frequencies, which will be more realistic.

4. Potential negative effects associated with following the 'method' or 'diet'.
Instead of putting forward scientific evidence and lines of argument, in the form of published articles, clinical trials and meta-analyses, all you have done is simply report on what experts from such or such a country have said without, however, ever adding anything yourselves. There is no reasoning here; only the enumeration of conclusions that other experts have arrived at, based on personal opinions or preferences, or even on financial interests, but none of this gives us a single shred of evidence.

To go back to your own words: '*the word of the* experts [which applies to the British Dietetic Association, the French Agency for Food Safety, etc.] *is of no value at all as far as scientific proof or public health are concerned.*' So please give us some scientific arguments, as I have been doing throughout this book.

My conclusion about the GREP-AEDN's fourth argument: In the absence of any scientific argument, we fall back upon the opinion of the 'experts'.

Postscript: I urge you to reconsider your stance or at the very least to argue it scientifically instead of resorting to this appalling attempt, full of contradictions and flawed lines of reasoning, to prove your case.

Letter to the French nutritionist, Jean-Michel Cohen

Dear Sir,

I am writing to you to express my disagreement with claims made in the various interviews you have given in Spanish newspapers which show that you have not examined this issue in any detail. Indeed, as I explain in a book based on the existing scientific bibliography, far from causing *'cardiovascular problems'*, a *'sharp rise in cholesterol'* or even *'breast cancer'*, as you state, ketogenic diets actually do the very opposite: they improve cholesterol, lower cardiovascular risk factors and the incidence of cardiovascular disorders and are used successfully to treat tumours.

Claims like this reveal a lack of scientific rigour and a fondness for fine words, when one would expect a real health professional, sincerely interested in his patients' wellbeing, to circulate truthful information by setting it out in such a way as to make it accessible to lay people.

There is another argument that raises a smile and shows that you cannot be such a good nutritionist as you claim. You say this: '*As a doctor, I have never had anything to complain about. I appear on television, I have good clients . . . I do admit that before I became well-known, I had more trouble getting results from my patients. Now that they see me as a celebrity, the pressure is greater, they feel that if they don't lose weight it's their fault as I have got nothing to prove.*' These claims only go to show that your weight-loss method is not good since it does not rely on a high quality scientific system, but rather on the patients' conviction and on their efforts to lose weight. In other words, once you are no longer there, their motivation disappears along with you so your patients put weight back on, proving that your method does not work. A sort of Pygmalion effect, but the other way round; your patients who believe in your expertise have to be up to the challenge, so that they don't let you down or let themselves down. I would love to know the long-term success rate for your diets, given that overall all diets have a 95 per cent failure rate after three years.

You also claimed that '*the problem with Dukan is not that there is too much animal protein but lots of things that are vital for good health get cut out. Cutting out potassium is very serious. If you do not eat fruit and vegetables, your potassium level drops and that has repercussions on many processes that go on in the body.*' On the one hand, all existing studies on ketogenic diets have never once recorded any cardiac alterations of any kind due to hypokalemia [potassium deficiency]. On the other hand, all these claims do is show that you are not acquainted with the Dukan method because for the whole diet the no-vegetable period lasts only, all in all, 3–7 days, depending on the individual. This is the first phase, and after this phase vegetables are then eaten on at least 3–4 days a week, and tomatoes in particular, which are one of the foods with the highest concentration of potassium. What is more, you are perhaps unaware that chicken and beef (220mg potassium per portion), cod, sardines, salmon (320mg potassium per portion), eggs (55mg potassium per portion), milk (350mg potassium per portion), yoghurt (400mg potassium per portion) and cheese (200mg potassium per portion) are just a few examples of foods of animal origin, among many others, that are equally rich sources of potassium. Do you still think that while eating this range of foods we would not get all the potassium we need, even without any fruit and vegetables? I will also add here that the epidemiological evidence of what many hunter-gatherer tribes eat, shows that low-carbohydrate, ketogenic diets are far better suited to our physiology than the diet you advocate.

Two further points before I conclude: if you had studied ketogenic diets in even the slightest detail, you would have learnt that this type of diet is good for our health and for our spirits, and that the ketogenic diet does not undermine either our health or our joie de vivre, as you claim. As for your claim that '*1,800 kilocalories are enough for all men to lose weight at a rapid pace and for all women to stabilize so this is a point where both genders converge'*, this shows, once again, that either you are trying to fool your patients, or that you know very little about basic maths (to set up a weight, age and calorie expenditure simulation) or thermodynamics. Moreover, in the same interview you claim that *'people over 25 who are fat will have lots of difficulty losing weight. I am optimistic for the youngest ones and moderately optimistic for those between 25 and 50.'* But why is this so, if you are saying that these 1,800 kcalories should solve all our problems? Your claims seem quite inconsistent to me, and you look at things superficially, basing your theories first and foremost on a priori knowledge (which is invalidated by the current state of scientific knowledge). I think that you should reconsider your position.

Postscript: Your claims are based on, mostly incorrect, a priori knowledge and you have not examined the Dukan Diet, ketogenic diets and their benefits in any detail. You treat issues superficially, while demonstrating that your scientific expertise is strangely far removed from what science tells us; the many articles published on the current benefits of ketogenic diets provide this information. To crown it all, the 'short-lived' success you have with your own patients owes nothing to your diet method being effective and is only due to a sort of Pygmalion effect, as you yourself admit in interviews. Unfortunately, there is little room for any science in all of this.

Letter to the French National Agency for Food Safety (ANSES) and to Miguel Ángel Martínez González, Professor of Preventive Medicine at the University of Navarra and obesity 'expert' ('few miracles in the Dukan Diet', on www.elpaís.com 11/09/2011)

Dear ANSES experts, dear Dr Martínez González,

I am writing to you because although I am aware that the opinion of experts is the worst evidence science can provide, the general public, on the other hand, does not realize this and puts its trust in what these so-called 'experts' say, whose justifications are usually limited to arguments such as: 'this is how it is', 'I am certain about it', 'you can believe me', 'I'm an expert in the field' and so on. The experts are said to be in possession of the truth, even though all truth (for the moment, until the opposite is proven) is based on serious scientific studies that undergo critical and methodological analysis. In this area, the claims published in the broadsheet *El País*, and supposedly inspired by your recommendations, appear to me inaccurate because they rest on erroneous assertions and/or ones without any scientific backing. So I would like to offer the following clarifications:

- If 8 out of 10 people doing the Dukan Diet put weight back on over the four years that follow, in all likelihood this is because they are not sticking to the lifetime rules of a weekly protein day and daily exercise. On the other hand, with regard to traditional diets, namely those that you and the other 'experts' recommend, 9.5 patients out of 10 put back on all the weight they've lost over the three years after their dieting. So the Dukan Diet has at least two successes in its favour: it is 15 per cent more successful compared with the standard diets, with an extra year without weight regain. Furthermore, if patients followed the advice they were given, I do not believe that they would put any weight back on. Unlike traditional diets, the Dukan method offers a safeguard that helps you stabilize. Whether people follow this advice or not is a different problem that has nothing to do with the diet as such but rather with each individual's willpower.

- With the Dukan Diet, protein intake is not three times greater than the recommended amount, nor does it result in a lack of fibre. But who decides what is recommended, and what is this based on? If we actually examine (as I have done in this book) the situation we find ourselves in because the current official recommendations are being applied, we see that from one country to another obesity has doubled or tripled and continues to be on the increase. These recommendations from the experts do not then seem to be working very well. And as we have also seen here, when we examine the studies available they show that ketogenic diets, and Dr Dukan's diet is one, are actually very good for our health insofar as they improve our lipid profile and cardiovascular risk, and help us prevent and fight cancer. Besides, they come close to the diet our ancestors ate, the hunter-gatherers from whom we get our genes and our physiology.

- Rather than merely claiming that this type of diet is likely to result in cardiac, kidney and liver problems, or even cancer, if we were to go by what you say, you ought to prove and publish such claims in scientific journals. Because for the time being, all serious publications in this field state the opposite – as we have clearly demonstrated in this book. All these casual assertions that are not backed up scientifically appear rather flimsy to me.

- I would like to say to Professor Martínez González that for a professional working in preventive medicine, who moreover is a university lecturer and obesity 'expert', he does not seem driven by the kind of critical mind one would expect from an academic. Moreover, as far as nutrition is concerned, he seems to know nothing of our evolution and origins; the hunter-gatherers whose genes we have inherited ate a ketogenic diet. Recent studies, as well as some that are not-so-recent, provide evidence that this type of low-carbohydrate diet is particularly effective in preventing and treating cancer and cardiovascular complaints. To my mind, for a university professor and obesity specialist not to mention a word of any of this is completely unheard-of. As for the following claim: '*This is all foreign to us. It's as if our genes recognized flavours from childhood, flavours that are so nice that they will fight to get them again*', this is a joke, because as we have seen, our genes are more accustomed to ketogenic diets than to any other. If Professor Martínez González had spent any time studying the matter and had bothered to update his scientific knowledge in this field, he would have read the works of Dr Pérez-Guisado from the University of Córdoba, which set out the benefits of ketogenic diets and highlight the usefulness of a Spanish Mediterranean ketogenic diet based on '*our nutritional values*', as he says. In other words, it is possible to eat a healthy, varied diet that is based on a Mediterranean lifestyle *while still being ketogenic* – i.e. one that is healthier than the excess carbohydrates the official bodies advocate. So, Professor, if you don't like the Dukan Diet, don't eat it but don't randomly criticize it and do acknowledge what is good about ketogenesis, at least what we currently know to be good scientifically. Finally, recognize that it is possible to eat a Mediterranean ketogenic diet that is healthier than the traditional Mediterranean diet since it only uses the healthy, useful elements from this diet.

Postscript: Once more, ANSES and Professor Martínez González prove to us that *it is not enough to claim to be an expert to be an expert* as their assertions are so devoid of scientific evidence and favour opinions that are of no value whatsoever from a scientific point of view. You do end up wondering how the National Food Safety Agency, which is meant to ensure that the French are healthy and eat well, can demonstrate such a lack of credibility and scientific thoroughness, and how university professors can be so adamant, so badly informed and so lacking in critical faculties.

CHAPTER NOTES

1. Why I wrote this book
'A study published in 2010 . . .': Elhayany A. *et al.*: A low-carbohydrate, Mediterranean diet improves cardiovascular risk factors and regulation of diabetes in obese patients suffering from diabetes mellitus type 2 (a randomized, year-long study) (*Diabetes Obes Metab.* 2010: 204–9)

'To my great regret . . . pilot studies': Schmidt M. *et al.*: The effects of a ketogenic diet on the quality of life of 16 patients with advanced cancer (pilot trial). *Nutr Metab*(Lond).2011;8(1):54

4. 50 questions
Question 2 – 'Conversely, it has been proven that . . .': 1. Eaton S.B. *et al.*: Evolution, body composition, insulin receptor competition, and insulin resistance. *Prev Med.* 2009; 49(4)283–5; 2. Lusting H. *et al.*: The toxic reality about sugar. *Nature.* 2012:482(7383):27–9; 3. Cordain L. *et al.*: Origins and evolution of the Western diet: health implications for the 21st century. *Am. J. Clin. Nutr.* 2005; 81(2):341–54; 4. O'Keefe J.H. Jr. *et al.*: Cardiovascular disease resulting from a diet and lifestyle at odds with our Paleolithic genome: how to become a 21st-century

hunter-gatherer. *Mayo Clin Proc.* 2004; 79(1):101–8; 5. Cordain L., et al.: Hyperinsulinemic diseases of civilization: more than just Syndrome X. *Comp. Biochem. Physiol. A Mol. Integr. Physiol.* 2003; 136 (1):95–112.

Question 6 – 'The benefits of calorie restriction in rodents and higher primates': Madrid J.A., Rol de Lama A.: Biological rhythms in nutrition and metabolism, A basic and clinical chronobiology.

Question 31 – 'The results show . . .' : Campillo Soto A., et al.: Preoperative very low-calorie diet and operative outcome after insertion of a gastric 'bypass'; a multi-centre randomized study / *Arch. Surg.* 2011 Nov; 146(11):1300–5.

BIBLIOGRAPHY

1. Dukan P., *The Dukan Diet Life Plan*, Hodder & Stoughton, 2011.
2. Dukan P., *The Dukan Diet*, Hodder & Stoughton, 2010.
3. Dukan P., *The Dukan Diet Recipe book*, Hodder & Stoughton, 2010.
4. Atkins R.C., *The New Atkins Diet*, Solar, 1995.
5. Levine I., 'Cancer among the American Indians and its bearing upon the ethnological distribution of the disease', *J. Cancer Res. Clin. Oncol.*, 1910; 9:422–435.
6. Orenstein A.J., 'Freedom of negro races from cancer', *Br. Med. J.*, 1923;2:342.
7. Prentice G., 'Cancer among negroes', *Br. Med. J.*, 1923;2:1181.
8. Brown G.M. *et al.*, 'The occurrence of cancer in an Eskimo', *Cancer*, 1952, 5:142–143.
9. Eaton S.B. *et al.*, 'Stone agers in the fast lane: chronic degenerative diseases in evolutionary perspective', *Am. J. Med.*, 1988;84:739–749.
10. Carrera-Bastos P. *et al.*, 'The western diet and lifestyle and diseases of civilization. Research Reports in Clinical', *Cardiology*, 2011;2:15–35.
11. Cordain L. *et al.*, 'Macronutrient estimations in hunter-gatherer diets', *Am. J. Clin. Nutr.*, 2000;72:1589–1592.

12. Hu Y. *et al.,* 'Stable isotope dietary analysis of the Tianyuan 1 early modern human', *Proc. Natl. Acad. Sci.,* USA, 2009; 106:10971–10974.

13. Richards M.P., 'A brief review of the archaeological evidence for Palaeolithic and Neolithic subsistence', *Eur. J. Clin. Nutr.,* 2002;56:16.

14. Ströhle A. *et al.,* 'Diets of modern hunter-gatherers vary substantially in their carbohydrate content depending on eco-environments: results from an ethnographic analysis', *Nutrition Research.,* 2011;31:429 – 435.

15. Campillo Soto Á., *El mono obeso: La evolución humana y las enfermedades de la opulencia: diabetes, hipertensión, arteriosclerosis, (The obese monkey: human evolution and the diseases of affluence: diabetes, hypertension, arteriosclerosis),* Crítica, 2007.

16. Grande Covián F., *Nutrición y Salud. Mitos, peligros y errores de las dietas de adelgazamiento (Nutrition and health. The myths, dangers and errors of slimming diets),* Temas De Hoy, 2007.

17. Pérez-Guisado J., 'Ketogenic diets: Additional benefits to the weight loss and unfounded secondary effects', *Arch. Latinoam Nutr.,* 2008;58(4):323–9.

18. Guyton A.C. & Hall J.E., *Textbook of Medical Physiology,* 9th ed., McGraw-Hill; 1996:927–952,1063–1077.

19. Frayn K., *Metabolic regulation,* Omega, 1998.

20. Castro del Pozo S., *Manual de patología general (Manual of general Pathology),* Masson, 2006.

21. López A. Rol de Lama, 'Ritmos biológicos en la nutrición y metabolismo' (Biological rhythms in nutrition and

metabolism), *Cronobiología Básica y Aplicada*, Editec@ Red SL, Madrid, 2006.

22. Béliveau R., *La Santé par le plaisir de bien manger (Health through the pleasure of eating well)*, Éditions Trécarré, 2009.

23. Campillo Soto Á., *Lo que su médico no sabe para salvarle la vida (What your doctor does not know about saving your life)*.

24. Klement R.J. *et al.*, 'Is there a role for carbohydrate restriction in the treatment and prevention of cancer?', *Nutr. Metab.* (Lond.), 2011 Oct. 26;8(1):75.

25. Chiu C.J. *et al.*, 'Does eating particular diets alter the risk of age-related macular degeneration in users of the Age-Related Eye Disease Study supplements?' *Br. J. Ophthalmol.*, 2009;93(9):1241–6.

26. Dessein P.H. *et al.*, 'Beneficial effects of weight loss associated with moderate calorie/carbohydrate restriction, and increased proportional intake of protein and unsaturated fat on serum urate and lipoprotein levels in gout: a pilot study', *Ann. Rheum. Dis.*, 2000;59:539–543.

27. Derr R.L. *et al.*, 'Association between hyperglycemia and survival in patients with newly diagnosed glioblastoma', *J. Clin. Oncol.*, 2009:27:1082–1086.

28. Stattin P. *et al.*, 'Prospective study of hyperglycemia and cancer risk'. *Diabetes Care*, 2007;30:561–567.

29. Seyfried T.N. & Shelton L.M., 'Cancer as a metabolic disease', *Nutr. Metab.* (Lond.), 2010;7:7.

30. Lee C. *et al.*, 'Fasting vs dietary restriction in cellular protection and cancer treatment: from model organisms to patients', *Oncogene*, 2011, 30:3305–3316.

31. Dashti H.M. *et al.,* 'Ketogenic Diet Modifies the Risk Factors of Heart Disease in Obese Patients', *Nutrition,* 2003; 19: 901–02.

32. Dashti H.M. *et al.,* 'Beneficial effects of ketogenic diet in obese diabetic subjects', *Mol. Cell. Biochem.,* 2007; 302:249–56.

33. Dashti H.M. *et al.,* 'Long term effects of ketogenic diet in obese subjects with high cholesterol level', *Mol. Cell. Biochem.,* 2006;286:1–9.

34. Brehm B.J. *et al.,* 'A Randomized Trial Comparing a Very Low Carbohydrate Diet and a Calorie-Restricted'; 'Low Fat Diet on Body Weight and Cardiovascular Risk Factors in Healthy Women', *J. Clin. Endocrinol. Metab.,* 2003;88: 1617–23.

35. Nobels F. *et al.,* 'Weight Reduction with a High Protein, Low Carbohydrate, Caloric Restricted Diet: Effects on Blood Pressure, Glucose and Insulin Levels', *The Netherlands Journal of Medicine,* 1989; 35: 295–302.

36. Gannon M.C. *et al.,* 'Effect of a high-protein, low-carbohydrate diet on blood glucose control in people with type 2 diabetes', *Diabetes,* 2004; 53: 2375–82.

37. Boden G. *et al.,* 'Effect of a low-carbohydrate diet on appetite, blood glucose levels, and insulin resistance in obese patients with type 2 diabetes', *Ann. Intern. Med.,* 2005; 142: 403–11.

38. Nuttall F.Q. *et al.,* 'The metabolic response to a high-protein, low-carbohydrate diet in men with type 2 diabetes mellitus', *Metabolism,* 2006; 55:243–51.

39. Volek J.S. *et al.,* 'Comparison of a Very Low-Carbohydrate and Low-Fat Diet on Fasting Lipids, LDL'; 'Subclasses,

Insulin Resistance, and Postprandial Lipemic Responses in Overweight Women', *J. Am. Coll. Nutr.*, 2004; 23:177–84.

40. Bisschop P.H. *et al.,* 'Dietary fat content alters insulin-mediated glucose metabolism in healthy men', *Am. J. Clin. Nutr.*, 2001; 73:554–59.

41. Yancy W.S. *et al.,* 'A low-carbohydrate, ketogenic diet to treat type 2 diabetes', *Nutr. Metab.*, 2005; 2:34.

42. Westman E.C. *et al.,* 'A Pilot Study of a Low-Carbohydrate, Ketogenic Diet for Obesity-Related Polycystic Ovary Syndrome', *J. Gen. Intern. Med.*, 2004;19(1S):111.

43. Mavropoulos J.C. *et al.,* 'The effects of a low-carbohydrate, ketogenic diet on the polycystic ovary syndrome: A pilot study', *Nutr. Metab.*, 2005; 2:35.

44. Major C.A. *et al.,* 'The effects of carbohydrate restriction in patients with diet-controlled gestational diabetes', *Obstet. Gynecol.*, 1998;9:600–04.

45. Farrés J. *et al.,* 'Revealing the molecular relationship between type 2 diabetes and the metabolic changes induced by a very-low-carbohydrate low-fat ketogenic diet', *Nutr. Metab.* (Lond.), 2010;7:88.

46. Caballero C. *et al.,* 'Obesidad, actividad e inactividad física en adolescentes de Morelos, México: un estudio longitudinal' (Obesity, physical activity and inactivity in adolescents in Morelos, Mexico: a longitudinal study), *Arch. Lat. Nutr.*, 2007, 57: 10–17.

47. Lambert E.V. *et al.,* 'Enhanced endurance in trained cyclists during moderate intensity exercise following 2 weeks adaptation to a high fat diet', *Eur. J. Appl. Physiol. Occup. Physiol.*, 1994; 69: 287–93.

48. Phinney S.D., 'Ketogenic diets and physical performance', *Nutr. Metabol.*, 2004; 1:1–7.

49. Sondike S.B. *et al.*, 'Low carbohydrate dieting increases weight loss but not cardiovascular risk in obese adolescents: a randomized controlled trial', *J. Adolesc. Health.*, 2000; 26: 91.

50. Phinney S.D. *et al.*, 'The human metabolic response to chronic ketosis without caloric restriction: physical and biochemical adaptation', *Metabolism*, 1983; 32: 757–68.

51. Fagan T.C. *et al.*, 'Effects of high protein, high carbohydrate, and high fat diets on laboratory parameters', *J. Am. Coll. Nutr.*, 1987; 6: 333–43.

52. Martin W.F. *et al.*, 'Dietary protein intake and renal function', *Nutr. Metab.*, 2005; 2:25.

53. Skov A.R. *et al.*, 'Changes in renal function during weight loss induced by high vs low-protein low-fat diets in overweight subjects', *Int. J. Obes.*, 1999; 23: 1170–77.

54. Knight E.L. *et al.*, 'The impact of protein intake on renal function decline in women with normal renal function or mild renal insufficiency', *Ann. Intern. Med.*, 2003; 138: 460–67.

55. Crowe F.L. *et al.*, 'Fruit and vegetable intake and mortality from ischaemic heart disease: results from the European prospective investigation into cancer and nutrition (EPIC)-Heart study', *Eur. Heart. J.*, 2011;32(10):1235–43.

56. Aggarwall B.B., *Healing Spices: How to Use 50 Everyday and Exotic Spices to Boost Health and Beat Disease*, Sterling, 2011.

57. Coy J. F., *Die neue anti-krebs-ernährung (The new anticancer diet)*, Gräfe und unzer, 2009.

58. Béliveau R., *Les Aliments contre le cancer (Anticancer foods)*, Éditions Trécarré, 2005.

59. Béliveau R., *Cuisiner avec les aliments contre le cancer (Cooking with anticancer foods)*, Éditions Trécarré, 2010.

60. Walenta S. *et al.*, 'High lactate levels predict likelihood of metastases, tumor recurrence, and restricted patient survival in human cervical cancers', *Cancer Res.*, 2000;60(4):916–21.

61. Fasano A., 'Zonulin and its regulation of intestinal barrier function: the biological door to inflammation, autoimmunity, and cancer', *Physiol. Rev.*, 2011;91:151–175.

62. Gonzalez F. *et al.*, 'Altered tumor necrosis factor alpha release from mononuclear cells of obese reproductive-age women during hyperglycemia', *Metabolism*, 2006;55:271–276.

63. Mantovani A. *et al.*, 'Cancer-related inflammation', *Nature*, 2008;454:436–444.

64. Mavropoulos J.C. *et al.*, 'Is there a role for a low-carbohydrate ketogenic diet in the management of prostate cancer?', *Urology*, 2006;68:15–18.

65. Fine E.J. *et al.*, 'Carbohydrate restriction in patients with advanced cancer: a protocol to assess safety and feasibility with an accompanying hypothesis', *Commun. Oncol.*, 2008;5:22–26.

66. Rieger J. *et al.*, 'The ERGO trial: A pilot study of a ketogenic diet in patients with recurrent glioblastoma', *J. Clin. Oncol.* (Meeting Abstracts), 2010;28:e12532.

67. Nebeling L.C. *et al.*, 'Implementing a ketogenic diet based on medium-chain triglyceride oil in pediatric patients with cancer', *J. Am. Diet. Assoc.*, 1995;95:693–697.

68. Nebeling L.C. *et al.*, 'Effects of a ketogenic diet on tumor metabolism and nutritional status in pediatric oncology patients: two case reports', *J. Am. Coll. Nutr.*, 1995, 14:202–208.

69. Schmidt M. *et al.*, 'Effects of a ketogenic diet on the quality of life in 16 patients with advanced cancer: A pilot trial', *Nutr. Metab.* (Lond.), 2011, 8:54.

70. Rossi-Fanelli F. *et al.*, 'Effect of energy substrate manipulation on tumour cell proliferation in parenterally fed cancer patients', *Clin. Nutr.*, 1991, 10:228–232.

71. Fine E.J. *et al.*, 'A pilot safety and feasibility trial of a reduced carbohydrate diet in patients with advanced cancer', *J. Clin. Oncol.*, 2011;29 (suppl; abstr e13573).

72. Masko E.M. *et al.*, 'Low-carbohydrate diets and prostate cancer: how low is "low enough"?' *Cancer Prev. Res.* (Phila), 2010, 3:1124–1131.

73. Freedland S.J. *et al.*, 'Carbohydrate restriction, prostate cancer growth, and the insulin-like growth factor axis', *Prostate*, 2008;68:11–19.

74. Tannenbaum A., 'The genesis and growth of tumors. II. Effects of caloric restriction per se', *Cancer Res.*, 1942, 2:460–467.

75. Zuccoli G. *et al.*, 'Metabolic management of glioblastoma multiforme using standard therapy together with a restricted ketogenic diet: Case Report', *Nutr. Metab.* (Lond.), 2010;7:33.

76. Ho V.W. *et al.*, 'A low carbohydrate, high protein diet slows tumor growth and prevents cancer initiation', *Cancer Res.*, 2011.

77. Otto C. *et al.*, 'Growth of human gastric cancer cells in nude mice is delayed by a ketogenic diet supplemented with omega-3 fatty acids and medium-chain triglycerides', *BMC Cancer*, 2008, 8:122.

78. Van Ness van Alstyne E. *et al.*, 'Diet studies in transplantable tumors. I. The effect of non-carbohydrate diet upon the growth of transplantable sarcoma in rats', *J. Med. Res.*, 1913:217–232.

79. Maurer G.D. *et al.*, 'Differential utilization of ketone bodies by neurons and glioma cell lines: a rationale for ketogenic diet as experimental glioma therapy', *BMC Cancer*, 2011;11:315.

80. Fine E.J., Miller A. *et al.*, 'Acetoacetate reduces growth and ATP concentration in cancer cell lines which over-express uncoupling protein 2', *Cancer Cell International*, 2009, 9:14:11.

81. Breitkreutz R. *et al.*, 'Effects of a high-fat diet on body composition in cancer patients receiving chemotherapy: a randomized controlled study', *Wien Klin Wochenschr*, 2005; 117:685–692.

82. Fearon K.C. *et al.*, 'Cancer cachexia: influence of systemic ketosis on substrate levels and nitrogen metabolism', *Am. J. Clin. Nutr.*, 1988, 47:42–48.

83. Beck S.A. *et al.*, 'Effect of insulin on weight loss and tumour growth in a cachexia model', *Br. J. Cancer*, 1989, 59:677–681.

84. Tisdale M.J. *et al.*, 'A comparison of long-chain triglycerides and medium-chain triglycerides on weight loss and tumour size in a cachexia model', *Br. J. Cancer*, 1988, 58:580–583.

85. Tisdale M.J. *et al.*, 'Reduction of weight loss and tumour size in a cachexia model by a high fat diet', *Br. J. Cancer*, 1987, 56:39–43.

86. Fearon K.C. *et al.*, 'Failure of systemic ketosis to control cachexia and the growth rate of the Walker 256 carcinosarcoma in rats', *Br. J. Cancer*, 1985, 52:87–92.

87. Magee B.A. *et al.*, 'The inhibition of malignant cell growth by ketone bodies', *Aust. J. Exp. Biol. Med. Sci.*, 1979, 57:529–539.

88. Conyers R.A. *et al.*, 'Cancer, ketosis and parenteral nutrition', *Med. J. Aust.*, 1979, 1:398–399.

89. Zhou W. *et al.*, 'The calorically restricted ketogenic diet, an effective alternative therapy for malignant brain cancer', *Nutr. Metab.* (Lond.), 2007, 4:5.

90. Tisdale M.J. *et al.*, 'Loss of acetoacetate coenzyme. A transferase activity in tumours of peripheral tissues', *Br. J. Cancer*, 1983, 47:293–297.

91. Young V.R., 'Energy metabolism and requirements in the cancer patient', *Cancer Res.*, 1977, 37:2336–2347.

92. Gambardella A. *et al.*, 'Different contribution of substrates oxidation to insulin resistance in malnourished elderly patients with cancer', *Cancer*, 1993, 72:3106–3113.

93. Conyers R.A. *et al.*, 'Nutrition and cancer', *Br. Med. J.*, 1979, 1:1146.

94. Waterhouse C. *et al.*, 'Gluconeogenesis from alanine in patients with progressive malignant disease', *Cancer Res.*, 1979, 39:1968–1972.

95. Permert J. *et al.*, 'Improved glucose metabolism after

subtotal pancreatectomy for pancreatic cancer', *Br. J. Surg.*, 1993, 80:1047–1050.

96. Yoshikawa T. *et al.*, 'Effects of tumor removal and body weight loss on insulin resistance in patients with cancer', *Surgery*, 1994, 116:62–66.

97. Makino T. *et al.*, 'Circulating interleukin 6 concentrations and insulin resistance in patients with cancer', *Br. J. Surg.*, 1998;85:1658–1662.

98. Marat D. *et al.*, 'Insulin resistance and tissue glycogen content in the tumor-bearing state'. *Hepatogastroenterology*, 1999, 46:3159–3165.

99. McCall J.L. *et al.*, 'Serum tumour necrosis factor alpha and insulin resistance in gastrointestinal cancer', *Br. J. Surg.*, 1992, 79:1361–1363.

100. Lundholm K. *et al.*, 'Insulin resistance in patients with cancer', *Cancer Res.*, 1978, 38:4665–4670.

101. Goodwin P.J. *et al.*, 'Insulin-like growth factor binding proteins 1 and 3 and breast cancer outcomes', *Breast Cancer Res. Treat.*, 2002, 74:65–76.

102. Venkateswaran V. *et al.*, 'Association of diet-induced hyper-insulinemia with accelerated growth of prostate cancer (LNCaP) xenografts', *J. Natl. Cancer Inst.*, 2007, 99:1793–1800.

103. LaPensee C.R. *et al.*, 'Insulin stimulates interleukin-6 expression and release in LS14 human adipocytes through multiple signalling pathways', *Endocrinology*, 2008, 149:5415–5422.

104. Shanmugam N. *et al.*, 'High glucose-induced expression of proinflammatory cytokine and chemokine genes in mono-cytic cells', *Diabetes*, 2003, 52:1256–1264.

105. Ely J.T. *et al.*, 'Glucose and cancer', *N. Z. Med. J.*, 2002, 115:U123.

106. Ikeda F. *et al.*, 'Hyperglycemia increases risk of gastric cancer posed by Helicobacter pylori infection: a population-based cohort study', *Gastroenterology*, 2009, 136:1234–1241.

107. Jee S.H. *et al.*, 'Fasting serum glucose level and cancer risk in Korean men and women', *JAMA*, 2005, 293:194–202.

108. Krone C.A. *et al.*, 'Controlling hyperglycemia as an adjunct to cancer therapy', *Integr. Cancer Ther.*, 2005, 4:25–31.

109. Maestu I. *et al.*, 'Pretreatment prognostic factors for survival in small-cell lung cancer: a new prognostic index and validation of three known prognostic indices on 341 patients', *Ann. Oncol.*, 1997, 8:547–553.

110. McGirt M.J. *et al.*, 'Persistent outpatient hyperglycemia is independently associated with decreased survival after primary resection of malignant brain astrocytomas', *Neurosurgery*, 2008, 63:286–291.

111. Koroljow S., 'Two cases of malignant tumors with metastases apparently treated successfully with hypoglycemic coma', *Psychiatr. Q.*, 1962, 36:261–270.

112. Seyfried T.N. *et al.*, 'Role of glucose and ketone bodies in the metabolic control of experimental brain cancer', *Br. J. Cancer*, 2003, 89:1375–1382.

113. Santisteban G.A. *et al.*, 'Glycemic modulation of tumor tolerance in a mouse model of breast cancer', *Biochem. Biophys. Res. Commun.*, 1985, 132:1174–1179.

114. Gatenby R.A. *et al.*, 'Why do cancers have high aerobic glycolysis?', *Nat. Rev. Cancer*, 2004, 4:891–899.

115. Masur K. *et al.*, 'Diabetogenic glucose and insulin concentrations modulate transcriptome and protein levels involved in tumour cell migration, adhesion and proliferation', *Br. J. Cancer*, 2011, 104:345–352.

116. Priebe A. *et al.*, 'Glucose deprivation activates AMPK and induces cell death through modulation of Akt in ovarian cancer cells', *Gynecol. Oncol.*, 2011, 122:389–95.

117. Demetrakopoulos G.E. *et al.*, 'Rapid loss of ATP by tumor cells deprived of glucose: contrast to normal cells', *Biochem. Biophys. Res. Commun.*, 1978, 82:787–794.

118. Fang J.S. *et al.*, 'Adaptation to hypoxia and acidosis in carcinogenesis and tumor progression', *Semin. Cancer. Biol.*, 2008, 18:330–337.

119. Gatenby R.A. *et al.*, 'Acid-mediated tumor invasion: a multidisciplinary study', *Cancer Res.*, 2006, 66:5216–5223.

120. Park H.J. *et al.*, 'Acidic environment causes apoptosis by increasing caspase activity', *Br. J. Cancer*, 1999, 80:1892–1897.

121. Williams A.C. *et al.*, 'An acidic environment leads to p53 dependent induction of apoptosis in human adenoma and carcinoma cell lines: implications for clonal selection during colorectal carcinogenesis', *Oncogene*, 1999,18:3199–3204.

122. Baumann F. *et al.*, 'Lactate promotes glioma migration by TGF-beta2–dependent regulation of matrix metalloproteinase-2', *Neuro. Oncol.*, 2009, 11:368–380.

123. Semenza G.L. *et al.*, 'Tumor metabolism: cancer cells give and take lactate', *J. Clin. Invest.*, 2008, 118:3835–3837.

124. Bonuccelli G. *et al.*, 'Ketones and lactate "fuel" tumor growth and metastasis: Evidence that epithelial cancer

cells use oxidative mitochondrial metabolism', *Cell Cycle*, 2010, 9:3506–3514.

125. Gatenby R.A. *et al.*, 'Cellular adaptations to hypoxia and acidosis during somatic evolution of breast cancer', *Br. J. Cancer*, 2007, 97:646–653.

126. Walenta S. *et al.*, 'High lactate levels predict likelihood of metastases, tumor recurrence, and restricted patient survival in human cervical cancers', *Cancer Res.*, 2000;60:916–921.

127. Jiang W. *et al.*, 'Dietary energy restriction modulates the activity of AMP-activated protein kinase, Akt, and mammalian target of rapamycin in mammary carcinomas, mammary gland, and liver', *Cancer Res.*, 2008, 68:5492–5499.

128. Azar G.J. *et al.*, 'Similarities of carbohydrate deficiency and fasting. Ketones, nonesterified fatty acids and nitrogen excretion', *Arch. Intern. Med.*, 1963, 112:338–343.

129. Klein S. *et al.*, 'Carbohydrate restriction regulates the adaptive response to fasting', *Am. J. Physiol.*, 1992, 262:E631–636.

130. LeRoith D., 'Can endogenous hyperinsulinaemia explain the increased risk of cancer development and mortality in type 2 diabetes: evidence from mouse models', *Diabetes Metab. Res. Rev.*, 2010, 26:599–601.

131. Choi N.C. *et al.*, 'Dose-response relationship between probability of pathologic tumor control and glucose metabolic rate measured with FDG PET after preoperative chemoradiotherapy in locally advanced non-small-cell lung cancer', *Int. J. Radiat. Oncol. Biol. Phys.*, 2002, 54:1024–1035.

132. Koppenol W.H. *et al.*, 'Otto Warburg's contributions to current concepts of cancer metabolism', *Nat. Rev. Cancer*, 2011, 11:325–337.

133. Sun Q. *et al.,* 'Mammalian target of rapamycin up-regulation of pyruvate kinase isoenzyme type M2 is critical for aerobic glycolysis and tumor growth', *Proc. Natl. Acad. Sci.,* USA, 2011;108:4129–4134.

134. Mamane Y. *et al.,* 'mTOR, translation initiation and cancer', *Oncogene,* 2006, 25:6416–6422.

135. Young C.D. *et al.,* 'Sugar and fat – that's where it's at: metabolic changes in tumors', *Breast Cancer. Res.,* 2008, 10:202.

136. Robey R.B. *et al.,* 'Is Akt the 'Warburg kinase'?-Akt-energy metabolism interactions and oncogenesis', *Semin. Cancer Biol.,* 2009, 19:25–31.

137. Robey R.B. *et al.,* 'Mitochondrial hexokinases, novel mediators of the antiapoptotic effects of growth factors and Akt', *Oncogene,* 2006, 25:4683–4696.

138. Pelicano H. *et al.,* 'Mitochondrial respiration defects in cancer cells cause activation of Akt survival pathway through a redox-mediated mechanism', *J. Cell. Biol.,* 2006, 175:913–923.

139. Warburg O., 'On respiratory impairment in cancer cells', *Science* 1956, 124:269–270.

140. Seyfried T.N. *et al.,* 'Cancer as a metabolic disease', *Nutr. Metab.* (Lond.), 2010;7:7.

141. Hanahan D. *et al.,* 'Hallmarks of cancer: the next generation', *Cell,* 2011;144:646–674.

142. Wen W. *et al.,* 'Dietary carbohydrates, fiber, and breast cancer risk in Chinese women', *Am. J. Clin. Nutr.,* 2009, 89:283–289.

143. Sieri S. *et al.,* 'Dietary glycemic index, glycemic load, and the risk of breast cancer in an Italian prospective cohort study', *Am. J. Clin. Nutr.,* 2007;86:1160–1166.

144. Melnik B.C. *et al.*, 'Over-stimulation of insulin/IGF-1 signaling by Western diet may promote diseases of civilization: lessons learnt from Laron syndrome', *Nutr. Metab.* (Lond.), 2011, 8:41.

145. Augustin L.S. *et al.*, 'Dietary glycemic index and glycemic load, and breast cancer risk: a case-control study', *Ann. Oncol.*, 2001, 12:1533–1538.

146. Pérez-Guisado J., 'Ketogenic diets and weight loss: basis and effectiveness', *Arch. Latinoam. Nutr.*, 2008;58(2):126–31. Review.

147. Pérez-Guisado J., 'C Athletic performance: muscle glycogen and protein intake', *Apunts. Medicina de l'esport*, 2008; 43:159. http://www.apunts.org.

148. Hannan M.T. *et al.*, 'Effect of dietary protein on bone loss in elderly men and women: the Framingham osteoporosis study', *J. Bone Miner. Res.*, 2000; 15: 2504–12.

149. Kerstetter J.E. *et al.*, 'The impact of dietary protein on calcium absorption and kinetic measures of bone turnover in women', *J. Clin. Endocrinol. Metab.*, 2005; 90: 26–31.

150. Dawson-Hughes B. *et al.*, 'Effect of dietary protein supplements on calcium excretion in healthy older men and women', *J. Clin. Endocrinol. Metab.*, 2004; 89: 1169–73.

151. Heaney R.P., 'Dietary protein and phosphorous do not affect calcium absorption', *Am. J. Clin. Nutr.*, 2000; 72: 758–61.

152. Heaney R.P., 'Excess dietary protein may not adversely affect bone', *J. Nutr.*, 1998, 128: 1054–57.

153. Ponce G.M. *et al.*, 'Ingesta de calcio y proteínas: relación con marcadores bioquímicos óseos en mujeres pre y

posmenopáusicas de Comodoro Rivadavia' (Protein and calcium intake: relationship with bone biochemical markers in pre and post-menopausal women in Comodoro Rivadavia) (Argentina), *Arch. Latinoamer. Nutr.*, 2006; 56: 237–243.

154. Gardner C.D. *et al.*, 'Comparison of the Atkins, Zone, Ornish, and LEARN diets for change in weight and related risk factors among overweight premenopausal women: the A TO Z Weight Loss Study: a randomized trial', *JAMA*, 2007;297(9):969–77.

155. Pérez-Guisado J. *et al.*, 'A pilot study of the Spanish ketogenic Mediterranean diet: an effective therapy for the metabolic syndrome', *J. Med. Food.*, 2011;14(7–8):681–7.

156. Pérez-Guisado J. *et al.*, 'Spanish ketogenic Mediterranean diet: a healthy cardiovascular diet for weight loss,' *Nutr. J.*, 2008;7:30

157. Paoli A. *et al.*, 'The ketogenic diet: an underappreciated therapeutic option?', *Clin. Ter.*, 2011;162(5):e145–e153.

158. Meckling K.A. *et al.*, 'Comparison of a low-fat diet to a low-carbohydrate diet on weight loss, body composition, and risk factors for diabetes and cardiovascular disease in free-living, overweight men and women', *J. Clin. Endocrinol. Metab.*, 2004;89(6):2717–23.

159. Popkin B.M. *et al.*, 'A comparison of dietary trends among racial and socioeconomic groups in the United States', *N. Engl. J. Med.*, 1996;335(10):716–20.

160. Meckling K.A. *et al.*, 'Effects of a hypocaloric, low-carbohydrate diet on weight loss, blood lipids, blood

pressure, glucose tolerance, and body composition in free-living overweight women', *Can. J. Physiol. Pharmacol.*, 2002;80(11):1095–105.

161. Jönsson T. *et al.*, 'A paleolithic diet is more satiating per calorie than a Mediterranean-like diet in individuals with ischemic heart disease', *Nutr. Metab.* (Lond.), 2010 Nov. 30;7:85.

162. Gannon M.C. *et al.*, 'Further decrease in glycated hemo-globin following ingestion of a LoBAG30 diet for 10 weeks compared to 5 weeks in people with untreated type 2 diabetes', *Nutr. Metab.* (Lond.), 2010 Jul. 29;7:64.

163. Yancy W.S. Jr *et al.*, 'A low-carbohydrate, ketogenic diet to treat type 2 diabetes', *Nutr. Metab.* (Lond.), 2005;2:34.

164. Westman E.C. *et al.*, 'The effect of a low-carbohydrate, ketogenic diet versus a low-glycemic index diet on glyc-emic control in type 2 diabetes mellitus', *Nutr. Metab.* (Lond.), 2008;5:36.

165. Haimoto H. *et al.*, 'Effects of a low-carbohydrate diet on glycemic control in outpatients with severe type 2 diabe-tes', *Nutr. Metab.* (Lond.), 2009;6:21.

166. Sasakabe T. *et al.*, 'Effects of a moderate low-carbohydrate diet on preferential abdominal fat loss and cardiovascular risk factors in patients with type 2 diabetes', *Diabetes Metab. Syndr. Obes.*, 2011;4:167–74.

167. Elhayany A. *et al.*, 'A low carbohydrate Mediterranean diet improves cardiovascular risk factors and diabetes control among overweight patients with type 2 diabetes mellitus: a 1–year prospective randomized intervention study', *Diabetes Obes. Metab.*, 2010;12(3):204–9.

168. Boden G. *et al.*, 'Effect of a low-carbohydrate diet on appetite, blood glucose levels, and insulin resistance in obese patients with type 2 diabetes', *Ann. Intern. Med.*, 2005;142(6):403–11.

169. Jabekk P.T. *et al.*, 'Resistance training in overweight women on a ketogenic diet conserved lean body mass while reducing body fat', *Nutr. Metab.* (Lond.), 2010;7:17.

170. Mutungi G. *et al.*, 'Dietary cholesterol from eggs increases plasma HDL cholesterol in overweight men consuming a carbohydrate-restricted diet', *J. Nutr.*, 2008;138(2):272–6.

171. Seyfried T.N. *et al.*, 'Targeting energy metabolism in brain cancer with calorically restricted ketogenic diets', *Epilepsia*, 2008;49 Suppl 8:114–6.

172. Seyfried T.N. *et al.*, 'Metabolic management of brain cancer', *Biochim. Biophys. Acta.*, 2011;1807(6):577–94.

173. Seyfried B.T. *et al.*, 'Targeting energy metabolism in brain cancer through calorie restriction and the ketogenic diet', *J. Cancer Res. Ther.*, 2009;5 Suppl 1:S7–15.

174. Greene A.E. *et al.*, 'Perspectives on the metabolic management of epilepsy through dietary reduction of glucose and elevation of ketone bodies', *J. Neurochem.*, 2003;86(3):529–37.

175. Vicente-Hernández M. *et al.*, 'Therapeutic approach to epilepsy from the nutritional view: current status of dietary treatment', *Neurología*, 2007;22(8):517–25.

176. Starbała A. *et al.*, 'The role of the ketogenic diet in the management of epilepsy', *Rocz Panstw Zakl Hig*, 2007;58(1):139–44.

177. Wheless J.W., 'Nonpharmacologic treatment of the

catastrophic epilepsies of childhood', *Epilepsia*, 2004;45 Suppl 5:17–22.

178. Kossoff E.H. *et al.*, 'A randomized, crossover comparison of daily carbohydrate limits using the modified Atkins diet', *Epilepsy Behav.*, 2007;10(3):432–6.

179. Kossoff E.H. *et al.*, 'Combined ketogenic diet and vagus nerve stimulation: rational polytherapy?', *Epilepsia*, 2007;48(1):77–81.

180. Kossoff E.H. *et al.*, 'A modified Atkins diet is effective for the treatment of intractable pediatric epilepsy', *Epilepsia*, 2006 Feb;47(2):421–4.

181. Porta N. *et al.*, 'The ketogenic diet and its variants: state of the art', *Rev. Neurol.* (Paris), 2009;165(5):430–9.

182. Kossoff E.H. *et al.*, 'A prospective study of the modified Atkins diet for intractable epilepsy in adults', *Epilepsia*, 2008;49(2):316–9.

183. Kossoff E.H. *et al.*, 'The modified Atkins diet', *Epilepsia*, 2008;49 Suppl 8:37–41.

184. Porta N. *et al.*, 'Comparison of seizure reduction and serum fatty acid levels after receiving the ketogenic and modified Atkins diet', *Seizure*, 2009;18(5):359–64.

185. Kossoff E.H. *et al.*, 'Will seizure control improve by switching from the modified Atkins diet to the traditional ketogenic diet?', *Epilepsia*, 2010;51(12):2496–9.

186. Miranda M.J. *et al.*, 'Danish study of a modified Atkins diet for medically intractable epilepsy in children: can we achieve the same results as with the classical ketogenic diet?', *Seizure*, 2011;20(2):151–5.

187. Vining E.P.G. *et al.*, 'A multi-center study of the efficacy

Bibliography

of the ketogenic diet', *Archives of Neurology*, 1998; 55:1433–37.

188. Tendler D. *et al.*, 'The effect of a low-carbohydrate, ketogenic diet on nonalcoholic fatty liver disease: a pilot study', *Dig. Dis. Sci.*, 2007;52(2):589–93.

189. Pérez-Guisado J. *et al.*, 'The effect of the Spanish ketogenic Mediterranean diet on nonalcoholic fatty liver disease: a pilot study', *J. Med. Food.*, 2011;14(7–8):677–80.

190. Noguchi Y. *et al.*, 'Ketogenic essential amino acids modulate lipid synthetic pathways and prevent hepatic steatosis in mice', *PLoS One*, 2010;5(8):e12057.

191. Campillo Soto Á. *et al.*, 'Preoperative very low-calorie diet and operative outcome after laparoscopic gastric bypass', a randomized multicenter study, *Arch. Surg.*

192. Al-Zaid N.S. *et al.*, 'Carbohydrate ketogenic diet enhances cardiac tolerance to global ischaemia', *Acta. Cardiol.*, 2007; 62:381–9.

193. Parks E.J. *et al.*, 'Carbohydrate-induced hypertriacylglycerolemia: historical perspective and review of biological mechanisms', *Am. J. Clin. Nutr.*, 2000; 71: 412–33.

194. Dashti H.M. *et al.*, 'Ketogenic diet modifies the risk factors of heart disease in obese patients', *Nutrition*, 2003; 19: 901–02.

195. Volek J.S. *et al.*, 'Fasting lipoprotein and postprandial triacylglycerol responses to a low-carbohydrate diet supplemented with N-3 fatty acids', *J. Am. Col. Nutr.*, 2000;19: 383–91.

196. Patsch J.R. *et al.*, 'Relation of triglyceride metabolism and

coronary artery disease: studies in the postprandial state',
Arterioscler. Thromb., 1992; 12: 1336–45.

197. Austin M.A. *et al.*, 'Hypertriglyceridemia as a cardiovascular risk factor', *Am. J. Cardiol.*, 1998; 81: 7B-12B.

198. Hellerstein M.K., 'Carbohydrate-induced hypertriglyceridemia: modifying factors and implications for cardiovascular risk', *Curr. Opin. Lipidol.*, 2002; 13: 33–40.

199. Hudgins L.C. *et al.*, 'Human fatty acid synthesis is stimulated by a eucaloric low fat, high carbohydrate diet', *J. Clin. Invest.*, 1996; 97: 2081–91.

200. Hudgins L.C., 'Effect of high-carbohydrate feeding on triglyceride and saturated fatty acid synthesis', *Proc. Soc. Exp. Biol. Med.*, 2000; 225: 178–83.

201. Yancy W.S. Jr *et al.*, 'A low-carbohydrate, ketogenic diet versus a low-fat diet to treat obesity and hyperlipidemia: a randomized, controlled trial', *Ann. Intern. Med.*, 2004; 140: 769–77.

202. Foster G.D. *et al.*, 'A randomized trial of a low-carbohydrate diet for obesity', *N. Engl. J. Med.*, 2003; 348: 2082–90.

203. Austin M.A. *et al.*, 'Atherogenic lipoprotein phenotype, a proposed genetic marker for coronary heart disease risk', *Circulation*, 1990; 82: 495–506.

204. Dreon D.M. *et al.*, 'A very-low-fat diet is not associated with improved lipoprotein profiles in men with a predominance of large, low-density lipoproteins', *Am. J. Clin. Nutr.*, 1999; 69: 411–18.

205. Campos H. *et al.*, 'Associations of hepatic and lipoprotein lipase activities with changes in dietary composition and low-density lipoprotein subclasses', *J. Lipid. Res.*, 1995; 36: 462–472.

206. Sharman M.J. *et al.*, 'Very low-carbohydrate and low-fat diets affect fasting lipids and postprandial lipemia differently in overweight men', *J. Nutr.*, 2004; 134: 880–85.

207. Westman E.C. *et al.*, 'Effect of a low-carbohydrate, ketogenic diet program compared to a low-fat diet on fasting lipoprotein subclasses', *Int. J. Cardiol.*, 2006; 110:212–16.

208. Dashti H.M. *et al.*, 'Beneficial effects of ketogenic diet in obese diabetic subjects', *Mol. Cell. Biochem.*, 2007; 302:249–56.

209. Dashti H.M. *et al.*, 'Long term effects of ketogenic diet in obese subjects with high cholesterol level', *Mol. Cell. Biochem.*, 2006;286:1–9.

210. Sondike S.B. *et al.*, 'Effects of a low-carbohydrate diet on weight loss and cardiovascular risk factors in overweight adolescents', *J. Pediatr.*, 2003; 42: 253–58.

211. Willi S.M. *et al.*, 'The effects of a high-protein, low-fat, ketogenic diet on adolescents with morbid obesity: body composition, blood chemistries and sleep abnormalities', *Pediatrics*, 1998;101:61–67.

212. Westman E.C. *et al.*, 'Effect of 6–month adherence to a very low carbohydrate diet program', *Am. J. Med.*, 2002; 113: 30–36.

213. Brehm B.J. *et al.*, 'A randomized trial comparing a very low carbohydrate diet and a calorie-restricted low fat diet on body weight and cardiovascular risk factors in healthy women', *J. Clin. Endocrinol. Metab.*, 2003;88: 1617–23.

214. Stern L. *et al.*, 'The effects of low-carbohydrate versus conventional weight loss diets in severely obese adults:

one-year follow-up of a randomized trial', *Ann. Intern. Med.*, 2004; 140:778–85.

215. Nobels F. *et al.*, 'Weight reduction with a high protein, low carbohydrate, caloric restricted diet: effects on blood pressure, glucose and insulin levels', *The Netherlands Journal of Medicine*, 1989; 35: 295–302.

216. Kopp W., 'Pathogenesis and etiology of essential hypertension: role of dietary carbohydrate', *Med. Hypotheses*, 2005; 64:782–87.

217. Lucas C.P. *et al.*, 'Insulin and blood pressure in obesity', *Hypertension*, 1985; 7: 702–06.

218. Muscelli E. *et al.*, 'Effect of insulin on renal sodium and uric acid handling in essential hypertension', *Am. J. Hypertens*, 1996; 9:746–52.

219. Rocchini A.P., 'Proceedings of the council for high blood pressure research, 1990: insulin resistance and blood pressure regulation in obese and non-obese subjects: special lecture', *Hypertension*, 1991; 17: 837–42.

220. Stamler J. *et al.*, 'Inverse relation of dietary protein markers with blood pressure. Findings for 10,020 men and women in the INTERSALT Study. INTERSALT Cooperative Research Group. International study of SALT and blood pressure', *Circulation*, 1996, 94: 1629–34.

221. Liu L. *et al.*, 'WHO-CARDIAC study group. Inverse relationship between urinary markers of animal protein intake and blood pressure in Chinese: results from the WHO cardiovascular diseases and alimentary comparison (CARDIAC) study', *Int. J. Epidemiol.*, 2002; 31: 227–33.

222. Lehninger Al., *Principios de bioquímica (Principles of biochemistry)*, Ediciones Omega; 1991: 531–557.

223. Okere I.C. *et al.*, 'Low-carbohydrate/high-fat diet attenuates cardiac hypertrophy, remodeling, and altered gene expression in hypertension', *Hypertension*, 2006; 48:1116–23.

224. Ratliff J.C. *et al.*, 'Eggs modulate the inflammatory response to carbohydrate restricted diets in overweight men', *Nutr. Metab.* (Lond.), 2008;5:6.

225. Mutungi G. *et al.*, 'Eggs distinctly modulate plasma carotenoid and lipoprotein subclasses in adult men following a carbohydrate-restricted diet', *J. Nutr. Biochem.*, 2010;21 (4):261–7.

226. Jarrett S.G. *et al.*, 'The ketogenic diet increases mitochondrial glutathione levels', *J. Neurochem.*, 2008;106:1044–51.

227. Haces M.L. *et al.*, 'Antioxidant capacity contributes to protection of ketone bodies against oxidative damage induced during hypoglycemic conditions', *Exp. Neurol.*, 2008; 211:85–96.

228. Ruskin D.N. *et al.*, 'Reduced pain and inflammation in juvenile and adult rats fed a ketogenic diet', *PLoS One*, 2009;4(12):e8349.

229. Servan-Schreiber D., *Anticancer. Prévenir et lutter grâce à nos défenses naturelles (Anticancer. Preventing and fighting it using our natural defences)*, Éditions Robert Laffont, 2007.

230. Calidad de la evidencia y grado de recomendación. (Quality of evidence and grade of recommendation) http://www.fisterra.com/guias2/fmc/sintesis.asp

231. Surh Y.J., 'Cancer chemoprevention with dietary phytochemicals', *Nature Reviews Cancer*, 2003: 3(10);768–780.

232. Poplawski M.M. *et al.*, 'Reversal of diabetic nephropathy by a ketogenic diet', *PLoS One*, 2011;6(4):e18604.

233. Kowluru R.A. *et al.*, 'Reversal of hyperglycemia and diabetic nephropathy: effect of reinstitution of good metabolic control on oxidative stress in the kidney of diabetic rats', *J. Diabetes Complications*, 2004;18(5):282–8.

234. Tonna S. *et al.*, 'Metabolic memory and diabetic nephropathy: potential role for epigenetic mechanisms', *Nat. Rev. Nephrol.*, 2010;6(6):332–41.

235. Yancy W.S. Jr, *et al.*, 'Acid-base analysis of individuals following two weight loss diets', *Eur. J. Clin. Nutr.*, 2007 Dec.;61(12):1416–22.

236. Dessein P.H. *et al.*, 'Beneficial effects of weight loss associated with moderated calorie/carbohydrate restriction, and increased proportional intake of protein and unsaturated fat on serum and lipoprotein levels in gout: a pilot study', *Ann Rheum Dis.*, 2000;59(7):539–43.

237. Reaven G.M., 'The kidney: an unwilling accomplice in syndrome X', *Am. J. Kidney Dis.*, 1997;30:928–31.

238. Reaven G.M., 'Insulin resistance: from bit player to centre stage', *CMAJ*, 2011;183(5):536–7.

239. Taubes G., *Good Calories, Bad Calories*, Anchor Books, 2007.

240. Masino S.A. *et al.*, 'Adenosine, ketogenic diet and epilepsy: the emerging therapeutic relationship between metabolism and brain activity', *Curr. Neuropharmacol.*, 2009;7(3):257–68.

241. Hartman A.L. *et al.,* 'The neuropharmacology of the ketogenic diet', *Pediatr. Neurol.,* 2007;36(5):281–92.

242. Gasior M. *et al.,* 'The anticonvulsant activity of acetone, the major ketone body in the ketogenic diet, is not dependent on its metabolites acetol, 1,2–propanediol, methylglyoxal, or pyruvic acid', *Epilepsia,* 2007;48(4):793–800.

243. Costantini L.C. *et al.,* 'Hypometabolism as a therapeutic target in Alzheimer's disease', *BMC Neurosci,* 2008;9 Suppl. 2:S16.

244. Reger M.A. *et al.,* 'Effects of beta-hydroxybutyrate on cognition in memory-impaired adults', *Neurobiol. Aging.,* 2004;25(3):311–4.

245. Mosconi L. *et al.,* 'Brain glucose hypometabolism and oxidative stress in preclinical Alzheimer's disease', *Ann. N.Y. Acad. Sci.,* 2008;1147:180–95.

246. Prins M., 'Diet, ketones, and neurotrauma', *Epilepsia,* 2008;49 Suppl 8:111–3.

247. Prins M.L., 'Cerebral metabolic adaptation and ketone metabolism after brain injury', *J. Cereb. Blood Flow Metab.,* 2008;28(1):1–16.

248. Maalouf M. *et al.,* 'The neuroprotective properties of calorie restriction, the ketogenic diet, and ketone bodies', *Brain Res. Rev.,* 2009 Mar.;59(2):293–315.

249. Lustig R.H. *et al.,* 'The toxic truth about sugar', *Nature,* 2012;482:27–29.

250. Campillo Soto Á., *Adelgazar para ejecutivos (Slimming for executives),* Plataforma editorial, 2012.

251. Lindstrom M., *Así se Manipula al Consumidor (Manipulate this consumer),* Gestión 2000, 2011.

252. Butryn M.L. *et al.*, 'Consistent self-monitoring of weight: a key component of successful weight loss maintenance', *Obesity* (Silver Spring), 2007;15(12):3091–6.

253. VanWomer J.J. *et al.*, 'Self-weighing promotes weight loss for obese adults', *Am. J. Prev. Med.*, 2009;36(1):70–3.

254. McGuire M.T. *et al.*, 'Long-term maintenance of weight loss: do people who lose weight through various weight loss methods use different behaviors to maintain their weight?', *Int. J. Obes. Relat. Metab.*, Disord. 1998;22 (6):572–7.

255. Karkhunen L. *et al.*, 'Psychobehavioural factors are more strongly associated with successful weight management than predetermined satiety effect or other characteristics of diet', *J. Obes.*, 2012; 2012:274068.

256. Bleich S.N. *et al.*, 'Impact of physician BMI on obesity care and beliefs', *Obesity* (Silver Spring), 2012, doi: 10.1038/ oby.2011.402.

257. Frisch S. *et al.*, 'A randomized controlled trial on the efficacy of carbohydrate-reduced or fat-reduced diets in patients attending a telemedically guided weight loss program', *Cardiovascular Diabetology*, 2009;8:36.

258. Miller W.C., 'Effective diet and exercise treatments for overweight and recommendations for intervention', *Sports Med.*, 2001;31(10):717–24.

259. Miller W.C., 'How effective are traditional dietary and exercise interventions for weight loss?', *Med. Sci. Sports Exerc.*, 1999;31(8):1129–34.